T0263794

Robotic Surgery

Editor

BERNARD J. PARK

THORACIC SURGERY CLINICS

www.thoracic.theclinics.com

Consulting Editor
M. BLAIR MARSHALL

May 2014 • Volume 24 • Number 2

ELSEVIER

1600 John F. Kennedy Boulevard • Suite 1800 • Philadelphia, Pennsylvania, 19103-2899

http://www.theclinics.com

THORACIC SURGERY CLINICS Volume 24, Number 2
May 2014 ISSN 1547-4127, ISBN-13: 978-0-323-29602-1

Editor: John Vassallo
Developmental Editor: Stephanie Carter

© 2014 Elsevier Inc. All rights reserved.

This periodical and the individual contributions contained in it are protected under copyright by Elsevier, and the following terms and conditions apply to their use:

Photocopying
Single photocopies of single articles may be made for personal use as allowed by national copyright laws. Permission of the Publisher and payment of a fee is required for all other photocopying, including multiple or systematic copying, copying for advertising or promotional purposes, resale, and all forms of document delivery. Special rates are available for educational institutions that wish to make photocopies for non-profit educational classroom use. For information on how to seek permission visit www.elsevier.com/permissions or call: (+44) 1865 843830 (UK)/(+1) 215 239 3804 (USA).

Derivative Works
Subscribers may reproduce tables of contents or prepare lists of articles including abstracts for internal circulation within their institutions. Permission of the Publisher is required for resale or distribution outside the institution. Permission of the Publisher is required for all other derivative works, including compilations and translations (please consult www.elsevier.com/permissions).

Electronic Storage or Usage
Permission of the Publisher is required to store or use electronically any material contained in this periodical, including any article or part of an article (please consult www.elsevier.com/permissions). Except as outlined above, no part of this publication may be reproduced, stored in a retrieval system or transmitted in any form or by any means, electronic, mechanical, photocopying, recording or otherwise, without prior written permission of the Publisher.

Notice
No responsibility is assumed by the Publisher for any injury and/or damage to persons or property as a matter of products liability, negligence or otherwise, or from any use or operation of any methods, products, instructions or ideas contained in the material herein. Because of rapid advances in the medical sciences, in particular, independent verification of diagnoses and drug dosages should be made.

Although all advertising material is expected to conform to ethical (medical) standards, inclusion in this publication does not constitute a guarantee or endorsement of the quality or value of such product or of the claims made of it by its manufacturer.

Thoracic Surgery Clinics (ISSN 1547-4127) is published quarterly by Elsevier Inc., 360 Park Avenue South, New York, NY 10010-1710. Months of publication are February, May, August, and November. Business and editorial offices: 1600 John F. Kennedy Boulevard, Suite 1800, Philadelphia, PA 19103-2899. Periodicals postage paid at New York, NY, and additional mailing offices. Subscription prices are $350.00 per year (US individuals), $453.00 per year (US institutions), $165.00 per year (US Students), $435.00 per year (Canadian individuals), $585.00 per year (Canadian institutions), $225.00 per year (Canadian and foreign students), $465.00 per year (foreign individuals), and $585.00 per year (foreign institutions). Foreign air speed delivery is included in all Clinics' subscription prices. All prices are subject to change without notice. **POSTMASTER:** Send address changes to Thoracic Surgery Clinics, Elsevier Health Sciences Division, Subscription Customer Service, 3251 Riverport Lane, Maryland Heights, MO 63043. **Customer Service (orders, claims, online, change of address): Telephone: 1-800-654-2452 (U.S. and Canada); 314-447-8871 (outside U.S. and Canada). Fax: 314-447-8029. Email:** journalscustomerservice-usa@elsevier.com **(for print support);** journalsonlinesupport-usa@elsevier.com **(for online support).**

Reprints. For copies of 100 or more, of articles in this publication, please contact Commercial Rights Department, Elsevier Inc., 360 Park Avenue South, New York, NY 10010-1710. Tel: 212-633-3874; Fax: 212-633-3820; E-mail: reprints@elsevier.com.

Thoracic Surgery Clinics is covered in *MEDLINE/PubMed (Index Medicus), EMBASE/Excerpta Medica, Science Citation Index Expanded (SciSearch®), Journal Citation Reports/Science Edition,* and *Current Contents®/Clinical Medicine.*

Contributors

CONSULTING EDITOR

M. BLAIR MARSHALL, MD
Associate Professor of Surgery, Georgetown
University School of Medicine; Chief, Division
of Thoracic Surgery, Department of Surgery,
Georgetown University Medical Center,
Washington, DC

EDITOR

BERNARD J. PARK, MD, FACS
Chief, Division of Thoracic Surgery,
Department of Surgery, Hackensack University
Medical Center, Hackensack, New Jersey

AUTHORS

ROBERT J. CERFOLIO, MD, MBA, FACS, FCCP
Professor of Surgery; Chief of Thoracic
Surgery; James H Estes Endowed Chair,
Lung Cancer Research, Birmingham,
Alabama

THOMAS A. D'AMICO, MD
Department of Surgery, Duke University
Medical Center, Durham, North Carolina

FEDERICO DAVINI, MD
Division of Thoracic Surgery, Department
of Cardio-Thoracic and Vascular Surgery,
University Hospital of Pisa, Pisa, Italy

OLIVIA FANUCCHI, MD
Division of Thoracic Surgery, Department
of Cardio-Thoracic and Vascular Surgery,
University Hospital of Pisa, Pisa, Italy

JENNIFER M. HANNA, MD, MBA
Resident in Cardiothoracic Surgery,
Division of Cardiovascular and Thoracic
Surgery, Department of Surgery, Duke
University Medical Center, Durham,
North Carolina

MAHMOUD ISMAIL, MD
Bereich Thoraxchirurgie, Charité
Universitätsmedizin Berlin, Berlin, Germany

KEMP H. KERNSTINE, MD, PhD
Professor and Chief, Division of Thoracic
Surgery, University of Texas Southwestern,
Dallas, Texas

DAVID LEHENBAUER, MD
4th Year General Surgery Resident, Parkland
Hospital, University of Texas Southwestern,
Dallas, Texas

BRIAN E. LOUIE, MD, MHA, MPH, FRCSC, FACS
Co-Director, Minimally Invasive Thoracic
Surgery Program; Assistant Program Director,
MIS Thoracic and Foregut Fellowships;
Director, Thoracic Research and Education,
Division of Thoracic Surgery, Swedish Cancer
Institute and Medical Center, Seattle,
Washington

FRANCA M.A. MELFI, MD
Chair of Multidisciplinary Center for Robotic
Surgery, Division of Thoracic Surgery,
Department of Cardio-Thoracic and Vascular
Surgery, University Hospital of Pisa, Pisa, Italy

ALFREDO MUSSI, MD
Chair of Division of Thoracic Surgery,
Department of Cardio-Thoracic and Vascular
Surgery, University of Pisa, Pisa, Italy

MARK W. ONAITIS, MD
Associate Professor, Division of
Cardiovascular and Thoracic Surgery,
Department of Surgery, Duke University
Medical Center, Durham, North Carolina

ALESSANDRO PARDOLESI, MD
Assistant, Division of Thoracic Surgery,
European Institute of Oncology, Milano, Italy

BERNARD J. PARK, MD, FACS
Chief, Division of Thoracic Surgery,
Department of Surgery, Hackensack
University Medical Center, Hackensack,
New Jersey

NABIL P. RIZK, MD
Assistant Attending, Thoracic Service,
Department of Surgery, Memorial
Sloan-Kettering Cancer Center; Associate
Professor of Cardiothoracic Surgery, Weill
Cornell Medical College, New York, New York

JENS C. RÜCKERT, MD, PhD
Bereich Thoraxchirurgie, Charité
Universitätsmedizin Berlin, Berlin, Germany

RALPH I. RÜCKERT, MD, PhD
Klinik für Chirurgie, Franziskus-Krankenhaus
Berlin, Akademisches Lehrkrankenhaus
der Charité Universitätsmedizin Berlin, Berlin,
Germany

INDERPAL S. SARKARIA, MD
Assistant Attending, Thoracic Service,
Department of Surgery, Memorial
Sloan-Kettering Cancer Center; Assistant
Professor of Cardiothoracic Surgery, Weill
Cornell Medical College, New York, New York

GARY S. SCHWARTZ, MD
Arthur B. and Patricia B. Modell Professor in
Thoracic Surgery, The Johns Hopkins Hospital,
Baltimore, Maryland

MARC SWIERZY, MD
Bereich Thoraxchirurgie, Charité
Universitätsmedizin Berlin, Berlin, Germany

GIULIA VERONESI, MD
Director, Lung Cancer Early Detection Unit,
Division of Thoracic Surgery, European
Institute of Oncology, Milan, Italy

BENJAMIN WEI, MD
University of Alabama, Birmingham, Alabama

STEPHEN C. YANG, MD
The Johns Hopkins Hospital, Baltimore,
Maryland

Contents

 Videos of Vats wedge resection of the left upper lobe, Isolation and resection of the tight upper vein, Isolation and resection of the right upper artery, Isolation and resection of the bronchus for the right upper lobe, Isolation of the vein from the middle lobe, Isolation and resection of the bronchus for the middle lobe, and Isolation and resection of the middle lobe arteries accompany this article

Retrospective series indicate that robot-assisted approaches to lung cancer resection offer comparable radicality and safety to video-assisted thoracic surgery or open surgery. More intuitive movements, greater flexibility, and high-definition three-dimensional vision overcome limitations of video-assisted thoracic surgery and may encourage wider adoption of robotic surgery for lung cancer, particularly as more early stage cases are diagnosed by screening. High capital and running costs, limited instrument availability, and long operating times are important disadvantages. Entry of competitor companies should drive down costs. Studies are required to assess quality of life, morbidity, oncologic radicality, and cost effectiveness.

Lobectomy with systematic lymph node sampling or dissection remains the mainstay of treatment of early stage non–small cell lung cancer. The use of video-assisted thoracic surgery (VATS) to perform lobectomy was first reported in 1992. Advantages of VATS include less trauma and pain, shorter chest drainage duration, decreased hospital stay, and preservation of short-term pulmonary function. However, VATS is characterized by loss of binocular vision and a limited maneuverability of thoracoscopic instruments, an unstable camera platform, and poor ergonomics for the surgeon. To overcome these limitations, robotic systems were developed during the last decades. This article reviews the technical aspects of robotic lobectomy using a VATS-based approach.

Robotic surgery is safe and efficient, with similar survival rates to the open and video-assisted thoracoscopic surgery (VATS) approaches. The surgeon can provide an R0 resection in patients with cancer. Technical modifications lead to decreased operative times and may improve the ability to teach. The capital cost, service contract costs, and equipment costs have to be carefully considered and studied, and patient selection is critical. There are few achievable benefits of using a robotic system compared with VATS when performing a sympathotomy for patients with hyperhidrosis or a pulmonary wedge resection for tissue diagnosis for patients with interstitial lung disease.

in all patients with myasthenia gravis in association with a resectable thymoma, typically Masaoka-Koga stages I and II.

THORACIC SURGERY CLINICS

RELATED INTEREST

Surgical Oncology Clinics of North America, Volume 22, Issue 1 (January 2013)
Laparoscopic Approaches in Oncology
James Fleshman, *Editor*
Available at http://www.surgonc.theclinics.com/

DOWNLOAD Free App!

Review Articles
THE CLINICS

NOW AVAILABLE FOR YOUR iPhone and iPad

Preface
Robotic Surgery

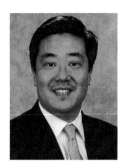

Bernard J. Park, MD, FACS
Editor

Over the past three decades there has been an explosion of advances in the field of minimally invasive surgery, including innovative new procedures, expanded indications, improved optics, and instrumentation. Perhaps one of the most radical and controversial recent advances has been the development of the master-slave, telerobotic surgical system and its widespread adoption for certain procedures, such as laparoscopic prostatectomy and hysterectomy.

Interestingly, telerobotic surgery was originally conceived and FDA-approved for closed chest cardiac surgery and yet it has not become widely adopted for revascularization or valve repair despite the fact that the robotic platform is unusually well-suited to a narrow surgical space such as the anterior mediastinum. Instead, the robotic platform has become the approach of choice for pelvic procedures in urology, gynecology, and colorectal surgery because of immediate, readily apparent technical advantages of three-dimensional vision and seven degrees of freedom of instrumentation.

Robotics has not had the same pace of implementation in general thoracic surgery perhaps because of skepticism regarding the interval benefit over nonrobotic VATS or laparoscopic procedures,

the learning curve involved in learning new techniques, and the stunning initial cost of the system. However, there has been interest building steadily in the role of telerobotics in the surgical management of thoracic disease as minimally invasive approaches fast become the standard of care.

This issue of the *Thoracic Surgery Clinics* attempts to review the technical aspects of several index thoracic procedures, such as anatomic lung resection, esophageal procedures, and approaches to mediastinal tumors. In addition, there is review of long-term results of robotic surgical treatment of early lung cancer and myasthenia gravis, as well as a candid look at the benefits and pitfalls of robotic technology in the field of minimally invasive surgery as a prelude to more in-depth assessments of the appropriate utilization of this complex technology.

Bernard J. Park, MD, FACS
Chief of Thoracic Surgery
Department of Surgery
Hackensack University Medical Center
Hackensack, NJ 07601, USA

E-mail address:
bpark@hackensackumc.org

http://dx.doi.org/10.1016/j.thorsurg.2014.02.013
1547-4127/14/$ – see front matter © 2014 Published by Elsevier Inc.

Robotic Thoracic Surgery
Technical Considerations and Learning Curve for Pulmonary Resection

Giulia Veronesi, MD

KEYWORDS

- Robotic surgery • Lung cancer • Video-assisted thoracic surgery

KEY POINTS

- Robot technology offers more intuitive movements, greater flexibility, and high-definition three-dimensional vision, which facilitates complex minimally invasive surgery with a potentially shorter learning curve than for video-assisted thoracic surgery (VATS).
- Robot technology for lung cancer resection and lymph node dissection seems to offer comparable radicality and safety to VATS and open surgery.
- Variables within robotic thoracic techniques include the number of incisions/arms, use of a utility incision for major lung resection, and use of CO_2 insufflation.

 Videos of Vats wedge resection of the left upper lobe, Isolation and resection of the tight upper vein, Isolation and resection of the right upper artery, Isolation and resection of the bronchus for the right upper lobe, Isolation of the vein from the middle lobe, Isolation and resection of the bronchus for the middle lobe, and Isolation and resection of the middle lobe arteries accompany this article at http://www.thoracic.theclinics.com/

The introduction of laparoscopic techniques was one of the major advances in twentieth-century surgery. Video-assisted thoracoscopic surgery (VATS) for lobectomy is an established approach to resectable lung cancer, characterized by reduced pain, fewer complications, and shorter postoperative stay compared with thoracotomy, although controversy persists regarding its oncologic equivalence to open surgery.[1–4] Furthermore, because of its limited field of view, restricted freedom of movement, and poor ergonomics, VATS lobectomy is a demanding procedure with a potentially long learning curve for surgeons and an approach that has not yet become the standard of care.

Robot-assisted surgery was introduced in the mid-1990s. One of its aims was to overcome the limitations of thoracoscopic surgery. Retrospective series of robotic lobectomy for lung cancer suggest that robot-assisted approaches offer comparable radicality and safety to VATS and open surgery. More intuitive movements, greater flexibility, and high-definition three-dimensional vision overcome limitations of VATS and may encourage wider adoption of robotic surgery for lung cancer, particularly as more early stage cases are diagnosed by screening. High capital and running costs, limited instrument availability, and long operating times are important disadvantages. However, a recent study suggests that rational multidisciplinary use of a robotic system coupled with optimization of postoperative patient management may improve cost effectiveness.[5] Entry of competitive alternatives into the marketplace should also drive down costs. Studies are required to assess quality of life, morbidity, oncologic radicality and cost

The author has nothing to disclose.
Lung Cancer Early Detection Unit, Division of Thoracic Surgery, European Institute of Oncology, Via Ripamonti 435, Milan 20141, Italy
E-mail address: giulia.veronesi@ieo.it

Thorac Surg Clin 24 (2014) 135–141
http://dx.doi.org/10.1016/j.thorsurg.2014.02.009
1547-4127/14/$ – see front matter © 2014 Elsevier Inc. All rights reserved.

effectiveness. This article focuses on technical considerations of incorporating the robotic system for minimally invasive thoracic surgery and the expected learning curve for major lung resection.

COMPONENTS OF THE TELEROBOTIC SURGICAL SYSTEM

The only commercially available robotic system for thoracic surgery is the da Vinci Surgical System (Intuitive Surgical, Sunnyvale, CA), a master/slave device consisting of four components (**Fig. 1**): (1) the robotic arms, (2) the surgeon's console, (3) the Insite vision system with a true three-dimensional high-definition endoscope providing a high-resolution binocular view of the surgical field, and (4) the EndoWrist instrument system capable of seven degrees of freedom and two degrees of axial rotation. The surgeon sits at the console, observes the operating field through binoculars, and manipulates the "master" instruments inserted through trocars placed through small, non–rib-spreading incisions. Manipulations of the master instruments are transmitted by the robot system into precise instrument movements inside the patient, with tremor filtration. The three-dimensional view largely compensates for the absence of haptic feedback.

TECHNIQUES FOR PULMONARY RESECTION

Techniques for robotic lobectomy vary in terms of the number of incisions and the use of a utility incision (VATS-based). The Milan group uses a four-arm system: three robot arm ports and a utility incision.[6] Other authors[7,8] in New York and Pisa started out using three arms, but subsequently adopted a four-arm technique. Dilewsky[9] and Cerfolio[10] use a four-arm, "total port" approach and make a utility incision only at the end of the procedure to insufflate the chest cavity with CO_2. The position of the utility incision (mainly to remove the surgical specimen) varies with surgeon preference. Veronesi[6] and Park[7] use a fourth intercostal space incision, whereas Dilewsky and coworkers[9] and Cerfolio and coworkers[10] introduced a lower supradiaphragmatic incision to reduce pain and facilitate the extraction of large tumors. Gharagozloo and coworkers[11] use a hybrid robotic-VATS technique. An important technical limitation of robotic surgery is that dedicated staplers, attachable to the robotic arms, are not yet available, so that the assistant surgeon has to maneuver staplers at the operating table. For the total port approach a fifth nonrobotic, assistant's port is required for passage of endovascular staplers.

PREOPERATIVE ASSESSMENT AND INDICATIONS

The indications for robotic lobectomy do not differ from those for VATS lobectomy. Patients must have adequate cardiopulmonary reserve, and lesions that are resectable by lobectomy or segmentectomy. However, as they gained experience,

A   **B**   **C**

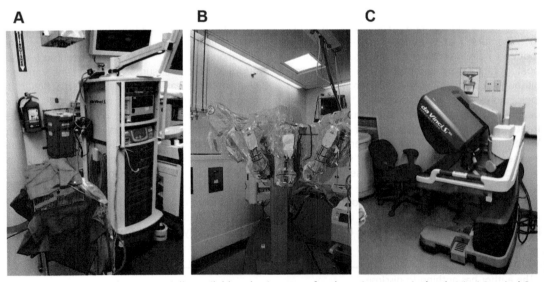

Fig. 1. The only currently commercially available robotic system for thoracic surgery is the da Vinci Surgical System (Intuitive Surgical, Sunnyvale, CA), a master/slave device consisting of four components: the robotic arms (*A*), the surgeon's console (*B*), the Insite vision system with a true three-dimensional high-definition endoscope providing a high-resolution binocular view of the surgical field (*C*). (*Courtesy of* Intuitive Surgical, Sunnyvale, CA; with permission.)

some robotic surgeons[9,10,12] have extended indications to advanced lung cancer after induction treatment, lymph node involvement, and centrally located lesions that require bronchial sleeve resection. Results seem to be satisfactory.[9,10] These extended resections require the skill and experience that can only be attained at centers performing large volumes of standard robotic lobectomies.

Standard staging procedures are performed and include computed tomography (CT), with contrast, of the chest, brain, and upper abdomen, and CT–positron emission tomography. For centrally located lesions, bronchoscopy is performed. CT-guided biopsy is performed in patients where a preoperative diagnosis is necessary, such as in patients with comorbidities, lesions with low level of suspiciousness for cancer, and centrally located lesions not amenable to VATS wedge resection.

SURGICAL TECHNIQUE
Patient Positioning and Port Placement

The patient is positioned in lateral decubitus and single-lung anesthesia achieved by a double-lumen endotracheal tube. The patient is prepared and draped with the arm down but if conversion to open surgery is necessary, the arm is moved up and a lateral muscle-sparing thoracotomy performed. The robot is positioned at the head of the patient (**Fig. 2**).

Using the four-arm technique, three port incisions and a 3-cm utility thoracotomy are made at the positions indicated in **Fig. 3**. The ports are standard for all lobectomies except that, on the right side, the camera port through the seventh intercostal space is in the mid-axillary line, whereas on the left side this port is moved 2 cm posteriorly (compared with the right) to avoid the heart obscuring vision of hilar structures. The utility incision is at the fourth intercostal space anteriorly.

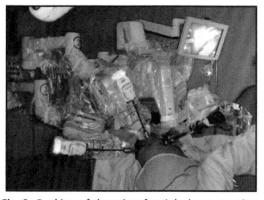

Fig. 2. Docking of the robot for right lung resection. (*Courtesy of* Intuitive Surgical, Sunnyvale, CA; with permission.)

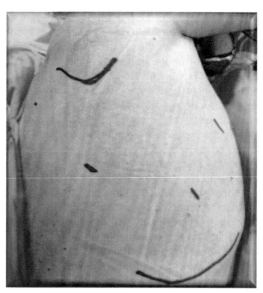

Fig. 3. Positions of ports and utility incision for robotic right lung resection according to the technique of the Milan group.[6] The utility incision is in the fourth intercostal space anteriorly. The camera port in the seventh or eighth intercostal space, mid-axillary line. The two posterior ports are in the ninth and seventh intercostal spaces, respectively.

Lesions without a preoperative diagnosis are first excised by standard VATS wedge resection followed by intraoperative frozen section examination. Small or deep undiagnosed lesions can be localized by multiple methods, such as methylene blue injection, wire localization, or by injecting ^{99}Tc-labeled sulfur colloid into the nodule under CT control up to 24 hours before surgery and use of an intraoperative gamma probe introduced through a port to precisely locate the "hot" nodule and hence guide the wedge resection (Video 1).[13]

Hilar Dissection

The lobectomy commences by isolating hilar elements using a hook or spatula and two Cadière graspers. The hook is manipulated by the right arm of the robot introduced through the utility thoracotomy for right-side dissections or through the posterior trocar in the eighth intercostal space for left-side lobectomies. One of the Cadière graspers (fourth robotic arm) is used to retract the lung and expose structures. The other grasper is manipulated by the left arm of the robot and used to grip structures during dissection: it is introduced through the utility thoracotomy for left-side lobectomies or through the posterior eighth intercostal space port for right-side lobectomies. When a hilar vessel or bronchus is ready to be surrounded with a vessel loop for stapler introduction, a third grasper is introduced (substituting the hook).

Vessels and the bronchus are sectioned using mechanical staplers introduced through a thoracoscopic port by the assistant surgeon after removal of a robotic arm. The pulmonary vein is usually the first structure to be isolated and divided (Video 2, right upper vein). If the lesion is in the right upper lobe, vein resection is followed by isolation of the branches of the pulmonary artery and sectioning (Video 3, right upper artery), followed by isolation of the bronchus and bronchus sectioning (Video 4, right upper bronchus). If the lesion is in the right lower lobe or left lung, after pulmonary vein sectioning, the bronchus is usually isolated and stapled before the artery. When performing middle lobectomy, the most favorable sequence is vein, bronchus, and artery (Video 5 middle vein, Video 6 middle lobe bronchus, and Video 7 middle lobe artery).

Fissure Completion and Lobe Removal

The fissure is completed by use of an endovascular stapler introduced by the assistant surgeon through one of the ports. The lobe is extracted through the anterior utility incision in an endoscopic pouch.

Mediastinal Lymph Node Dissection

Although suspicious lymph nodes are usually removed before lobectomy, radical lymph node dissection is performed after lobectomy using the same technique as in open surgery.[14] Paratracheal lymph node dissection is performed on the right side usually without azygos vein division. The mediastinal pleura between the superior vena cava and the azygos vein is incised. The lymph nodes, together with the fatty soft tissue of the region of the Barety space, are removed en bloc using a hook and Cadière grasper. In patients with large quantities of mediastinal fat or very large lymph nodes a harmonic scalpel may be used.

The nodes of the subcarinal station are removed after resection of the pulmonary ligament and retraction of the lung toward the anterior mediastinum to expose the posterior mediastinum. Bronchial arteries can usually be avoided thanks to good visibility; if not they are simply coagulated. A clip is not usually required. A single pleural drain is positioned in one of the small anterior incisions at the end of the operation.

POSTOPERATIVE CARE

Intensive care is not normally necessary. Patients are typically awakened in the operating room soon after the conclusion of surgery and brought to the ward. Chest radiograph and blood tests are done in the immediate postsurgical period. Patients are mobilized and start pulmonary rehabilitation on the first postoperative day; the vesical catheter is removed on the same day if diuresis is adequate (>30 mL/h) and there are no other contraindications. The drain is removed when less than 350 to 400 mL has accumulated over the preceding 24 hours (175 mL over 12 hours) and air leaks are absent. Discharge is possible on the same day as drain removal (third postoperative day at the earliest). In the event of prolonged air leakage, a Heimlich valve is attached to the chest tube, and discharge planned for the fifth postoperative day in the absence of further contraindications.

REPORTED CLINICAL OUTCOMES

Table 1 summarizes surgical technique and outcomes in studies reporting on 30 or more robotic lung lobectomies. Melfi and Mussi[8] reported on 107 robotic lobectomies with lymphadenectomy performed in "good-risk" oncologic patients, with good results in terms of complications, number of conversions, and duration of surgery. The feasibility and safety of the new technique was established by other early publications including those by Park and colleagues[7] on 34 lung cancer lobectomies published in 2006, and Gharagozloo and coworkers[11] who reported on 100 consecutive cases using a hybrid, two-phase procedure (robotic vascular, hilar, and mediastinal dissection, followed by VATS lobectomy). Veronesi and colleagues[6] reported the first comparison of open muscle-sparing thoracotomy with robotic lobectomy using a novel four-arm technique. Propensity scores for preoperative variables were used to match the 54 robotic patients with 54 that underwent open surgery. Hospital stay was shorter in the robotic group, but operating times were longer; however, after the first tertile of cases, the duration of surgery reduced significantly. It was concluded that robotic lobectomy with lymph node dissection was practicable and safe.

In 2011, Dylewski and colleagues[9] reported on 200 lung robotic resections using a novel approach in which pulmonary resection was performed through the ports only, without a utility incision, and pneumothorax was induced by CO_2 insufflation. At the end of the procedure the specimen was extracted by a subcostal transdiaphragmatic approach, and the diaphragm subsequently repaired. Median duration of surgery was short at 100 minutes (range, 30–279) and median stay was 3 days. However, the readmission rate was high (10%) usually for effusion, requiring drainage, or postoperative pneumothorax. Cerfolio and colleagues's[10] 2011 paper reported retrospectively

Table 1
Summary of results of publications on robotic lung resections (>30 cases)

Study, Year	Number of Patients	Mean Operating Time (min)	Mean Postoperative Stay (d)	Postoperative Complication Rate (%)	Mortality (%)	Conversion (%)
Robotic lobectomy/segmentectomy with utility incision						
Park et al,[7] 2006	30	218	4.5	26	0	12
Melfi & Mussi,[8] 2008	107	220	5	NA	1	NA
Gharagozloo et al,[11] 2009	100	216	4	21	3	13
Veronesi et al,[6] 2010	54	224	4.5	20	0	9.4
Park et al,[13] 2012	325	210	5	25	0.1	8
Veronesi et al,[16] 2011	91	213	5	20	0	10
Robotic lobectomy/segmentectomy without utility incision						
Dylewski et al,[9] 2011	165/35	90	3	26	0	1.5
Cerfolio et al,[10] 2011	106/16	132	2	27	0	10

on a consecutive series of 107 completely portal (no utility incision) four-arm lobectomies, in comparison with 318 propensity-matched cases treated by nerve- and rib-sparing thoracotomy. The robotic group had lower morbidity and mortality, improved mental quality of life, and shorter stay. The authors changed their robotic technique during the experience, adding a fourth robotic arm for retraction, a vessel loop to guide the stapler, and CO_2 insufflation. These changes were associated with reduced operating times and conversions. The authors commented that their robotic series did not exclude cases with larger tumors, N1 disease, or previous chemoradiation, and that many of these patients would not have been offered VATS (usually reserved for T1-T2 cases). These changes amount to enlarged indications for minimally invasive lung cancer resection, because the robotic approach allows R0 resection (complete with disease-free margins) of tumors up to 9.4 cm. Park et al[13] repeated long term results of 325 patients that underwent robotic lobectomy per lung cancer with results comparable to those obtained after VATS or open approach.

LEARNING AND TRAINING

Learning may be more rapid with robotic surgery than laparoscopic surgery. Chang and colleagues[14] found that after 8 to 10 hours of robotic training, intracorporeal knot-tying was shorter with the robot than by laparoscopy among surgeons who had variable laparoscopic experience but no robotic experience. There was further improvement after 14 hours of training. Hernandez and colleagues[15] divided surgeons into two groups according to laparoscopic experience and had

them perform five synthetic small bowel anastomoses using the da Vinci robot. Differences between the first and fifth attempts were assessed by time taken, the Objective Structured Assessment of Surgical Skills scale,[17] and the da Vinci motion analysis software. Surgeons quickly became proficient with the robotic system, irrespective of whether they had prior laparoscopic experience. Other studies have addressed learning for robotic surgery[18,19]; however, information on learning for robotic lung lobectomy is limited.[8,11,16,20,21]

Melfi and Mussi[8] did not provide a learning curve for their report on 107 robotic lobectomies, but suggested that a minimum of 20 operations was necessary for surgeons and nurses to attain proficiency. They also emphasized that procedure standardization was fundamental for good results. Based on operating times and hospital stay Gharagozloo and colleagues[11] suggested that 20 operations were required to attain sufficient skill.

Of the 91 consecutive robotic lung lobectomies reported by Veronesi and colleagues[16] the first 18 had significantly longer median operating times and postoperative hospitalization times than the later cases, whereas conversion and complication rates reduced nonsignificantly in the later cases (**Fig. 4**). The authors suggested that about 20 operations were required for a surgeon experienced in open thoracic surgery (but not VATS) to achieve competence with robotic lobectomy.

The 2011 paper by Jang and colleagues[20] retrospectively compared robot-assisted lobectomy for non–small cell lung cancer in 40 patients with results for first 40 patients treated by VATS, and also the most recent VATS series. There were no conversions in the robotic group, whereas conversions were 8% and 5%, respectively, in the initial

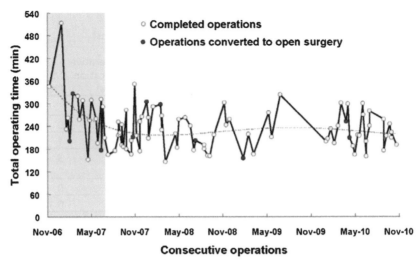

Fig. 4. Learning curve derived from analysis of operating times for robotic lung lobectomies. (*From* Veronesi G, Agoglia B, Melfi F, et al. Experience with robotic lobectomy for lung. Innovations (Phila) 2011;6(6):358; with permission.)

and mature VATS groups. Intraoperative bleeding was less in the robotic than the initial VATS group (219 vs 374 mL; P = .017), and median postoperative stay was significantly shorter (6 vs 9 days; $P<.001$). These data therefore suggest shorter learning for robotic than VATS lobectomy. **Table 2** shows estimates from recent publications of the number of operations required to achieve proficiency with VATS lobectomy and robotic lobectomy.[8,11,16,20–26]

Table 2		
Number of operations considered necessary to attain adequate skill in lung lobectomy by VATS and robotic approaches		
Study, Year	Lung Operation	No. of Operations Required
Melfi & Mussi,[8] 2008	Robotic lobectomy	20
Gharagozloo et al,[11] 2009	Robotic lobectomy	20
Veronesi et al,[6] 2010	Robotic lobectomy	20
Jang et al,[20] 2011	Robotic lobectomy	6
Lee et al,[22] 2009	VATS lobectomy	30–50
Belgers et al,[23] 2010	VATS lobectomy	25–30
Petersen & Hansen,[24] 2010	VATS lobectomy	50

Because robotic surgery is rapidly gaining ground, specialist training programs may be advisable to help surgeons acquire the necessary skills. Kajiwara and colleagues[21] proposed a program using pigs to train thoracic surgeons in robotic techniques. Milan investigators proposed a program not involving animal sacrifice[16] but using technical and clinical mentors to cover the basics of the robot and its instruments, surgical procedures, and "tricks of the trade." The program also includes lectures, case discussions, observation of live surgery, and hands-on sessions using the MIMIC 37 software[25] and da Vinci Si double consoles.

SUMMARY

Telerobotic surgery systems confer several technical advantages over traditional manual videothoracoscopic surgery, such as more intuitive movements, greater flexibility, and high-definition three-dimensional optics. These technologic advances can overcome certain limitations of VATS and may encourage wider adoption of minimally invasive approaches for the surgical treatment of thoracic disease. There are variations in robotic techniques for anatomic lung resection in terms of number of incisions, use of a utility incision versus a total port approach, and use of CO_2 insufflation. However, regardless of technique there is growing evidence to indicate that robot-assisted approaches to minimally invasive lung resection offer comparable radicality and safety to VATS and open surgery. Ongoing prospective studies are required to assess for differences between robotic, VATS, and open approaches with respect to long-term outcomes, oncologic efficacy, quality of life, and cost implications.

SUPPLEMENTARY DATA

Videos related to this article can be found online at http://dx.doi.org/10.1016/j.thorsurg.2014.02.009.

REFERENCES

1. Boffa DJ, Kosinski AS, Paul S, et al. Lymph node evaluation by open or video-assisted approaches in 11,500 anatomic lung cancer resections. Ann Thorac Surg 2012;94(2):347–53.
2. Swanson SJ, Herndon JE II, D'Amico TA, et al. Video-assisted thoracic surgery lobectomy: report of CALGB 39802-a prospective, multi-institution feasibility study. J Clin Oncol 2007;25:4993–7.
3. Whitson BA, D'Cunha J, Andre RS, et al. Thoracoscopic versus thoracotomy approaches to lobectomy: differential impairment of cellular immunity. Ann Thorac Surg 2008;86:1735–44.
4. Licht PB, Jørgensen OD, Ladegaard L, et al. A national study of nodal upstaging after thoracoscopic versus open lobectomy for clinical stage I lung cancer. Ann Thorac Surg 2013;96:943–9. http://dx.doi.org/10.1016/j.athoracsur.2013.04.011.
5. Park BJ, Flores RM. Cost comparison of robotic, video-assisted thoracic surgery and thoracotomy approaches to pulmonary lobectomy. Thorac Surg Clin 2008;18:297–300.
6. Veronesi G, Galetta D, Maisonneuve P, et al. Four-arm robotic lobectomy for the treatment of early-stage lung cancer. J Thorac Cardiovasc Surg 2010;140(1):19–25.
7. Park BJ, Flores RM, Rusch VW. Robotic assistance for video-assisted thoracic surgical lobectomy: technique and initial results. J Thorac Cardiovasc Surg 2006;131(1):54–9.
8. Melfi FM, Mussi A. Robotically assisted lobectomy: learning curve and complications. Thorac Surg Clin 2008;18:289–95. http://dx.doi.org/10.1016/j.thorsurg.2008.06.001, vi–vii.
9. Dylewski MR, Ohaeto AC, Pereira JF. Pulmonary resection using a total endoscopic robotic video-assisted approach. Semin Thorac Cardiovasc Surg 2011;23(1):36–42. http://dx.doi.org/10.1053/j.semtcvs.2011.01.005.
10. Cerfolio RJ, Bryant AS, Skylizard L, et al. Initial consecutive experience of completely portal robotic pulmonary resection with 4 arms. J Thorac Cardiovasc Surg 2011;142(4):740–6. http://dx.doi.org/10.1016/j.jtcvs.2011.07.022.
11. Gharagozloo F, Margolis M, Tempesta B, et al. Robot-assisted lobectomy for early-stage lung cancer: report of 100 consecutive cases. Ann Thorac Surg 2009;88(2):380–4. http://dx.doi.org/10.1016/j.athoracsur.2009.04.039.
12. Spaggiari L, Galetta D. Pneumonectomy for lung cancer: a further step in minimally invasive surgery. Ann Thorac Surg 2011;91(3):e45–7.
13. Park BJ, Melfi F, Mussi A, et al. Robotic lobectomy for non-small cell lung cancer (NSCLC): long-term oncologic results. J Thorac Cardiovasc Surg 2012;143(2):383–9.
14. Chang L, Satava RM, Pellegrini CA, et al. Robotic surgery: identifying the learning curve through objective measurement of skill. Surg Endosc 2003;17(11):1744–8.
15. Hernandez J, Bann S, Munz K, et al. Qualitative and quantitative analysis of the learning curve of a simulated task on the da Vinci system. Surg Endosc 2004;18:372–8.
16. Veronesi G, Agoglia B, Melfi F, et al. Experience with robotic lobectomy for lung. Innovations (Phila) 2011;6(6):355–60.
17. Martin J, Regehr G, Reznick R, et al. Objective structured assessment of technical skills (OSATS) for surgical residents. Br J Surg 1997;84:273–8.
18. Moorthy K, Munz Y, Dosis A, et al. Dexterity enhancement with robotic surgery. Surg Endosc 2004;18:790–5.
19. Maniar HS, Council ML, Prasad SM, et al. Comparison of skill training with robotic systems and traditional endoscopy: implications on training and adoption. J Surg Res 2005;125:23–9.
20. Jang HJ, Lee HS, Park SY, et al. Comparison of the early robot-assisted lobectomy experience to video-assisted thoracic surgery lobectomy for lung cancer: a single-institution case series matching study. Innovations (Phila) 2011;6(5):305–10.
21. Kajiwara N, Kakihana M, Usuda J, et al. Training in robotic surgery using the da Vinci Surgical System for left pneumonectomy and lymph node dissection in an animal model. Ann Thorac Cardiovasc Surg 2011;17(5):446–53.
22. Lee HS, Nam BH, Zo JI. Learning curves for video-assisted thoracic surgery lobectomy in non-small cell lung cancer. 89th Annual Meeting of AATS. Boston, May 9–13, 2009. Available at: http://www.aats.org/annualmeeting/Abstracts/2009/15.html. Accessed July 3, 2013.
23. Belgers EH, Siebenga J, Bosch AM, et al. Complete video-assisted thoracoscopic surgery lobectomy and its learning curve. A single center study introducing the technique in The Netherlands. Interact Cardiovasc Thorac Surg 2010;10:176–80.
24. Petersen RH, Hansen HJ. Learning thoracoscopic lobectomy. Eur J Cardiothorac Surg 2010;37:516–20.
25. Lerner MA, Ayalew M, Peine WJ, et al. Does training on a virtual reality robotic simulator improve performance on the da Vinci Surgical System? J Endourol 2010;24(3):467–72.
26. McKenna R. Complications and learning curves for video-assisted thoracic surgery lobectomy. Thorac Surg Clin 2008;18:275–80.

VATS-based Approach for Robotic Lobectomy

Franca M.A. Melfi, MD*, Olivia Fanucchi, MD, Federico Davini, MD, Alfredo Mussi, MD

KEYWORDS

• Robotic • Lobectomy • Lung cancer • Minimally invasive surgery • NSCLC

KEY POINTS

- Robotic lobectomy should not be considered experimental, but an accepted minimally invasive thoracic surgical technique.
- The robotic system provides stereoscopic binocular vision allowing the surgeon depth perception and high optical resolution. Three-dimensional imaging is one of the advantages over traditional VATS images, which are two-dimensionally displayed in the monitor.
- Magnified video imaging up to 10 times the actual size is helpful to delineate anatomic relationships and is idea for narrow spaces, such as the anterior mediastinum or pelvis.
- Robotic instruments reproduce the human hand's degrees of freedom, which are lost during VATS surgery.
- Future evaluation of differences among robotic, VATS, and thoracotomy approaches to thoracic diseases is warranted in terms of long-term outcomes.

INTRODUCTION

Lobectomy with systematic lymph node sampling or dissection remains the mainstay of treatment of early stage non–small cell lung cancer (NSCLC) since the Lung Cancer Study Group performed the only randomized prospective study comparing lobectomy with limited resection and showed that lobectomy had lower local recurrence and a trend toward superior survival.[1] Before the 1990s the only surgical approach to lobectomy was thoracotomy. In 1992, Lewis and colleagues[2] first reported the use of video-assisted thoracic surgery (VATS) to perform 40 lobectomies. Several subsequent studies demonstrated several advantages of VATS: less trauma and pain,[3] shorter chest drainage duration, decreased hospital stay,[4,5] and preservation of short-term pulmonary function.[6] However, VATS is characterized by loss of binocular vision and a limited maneuverability of thoracoscopic instruments, an unstable camera platform, and poor ergonomics for the surgeon. To overcome these limitations, robotic systems were developed during the last decades. The Automated Endoscopic System for Optimal Positioning was the first arm approved by the US Food and Drug Administration to be used in laparoscopic surgery.[7] Subsequently, the same company (Computer Motion Inc, Goleta, CA) developed the ZEUS system to assist surgeons in minimally invasive surgery.[8–10] In parallel, the da Vinci Surgical System was developed by Intuitive Surgical (Sunnyvale, CA) and approved by the Food and Drug Administration for laparoscopy, thoracoscopy, and intracardiac mitral valve repair. Currently, the da Vinci Surgical System is the only commercially available surgical system applied in a wide range of surgical procedures. This article reviews the technical aspects of robotic lobectomy using a VATS-based approach.

Disclosure: Franca Melfi is an official proctoring of Intuitive. The other authors have nothing to disclose.
Division of Thoracic Surgery, Department of Cardio-Thoracic and Vascular Surgery, University Hospital of Pisa, Via Paraisa 2, Pisa 56124, Italy
* Corresponding author. Robotic Multidisciplinary Center for Surgery, University Hospital of Pisa, Via Paraisa 2, Pisa 56124, Italy.
E-mail address: franca.mamelfi@gmail.com

1547-4127/14/$ – see front matter © 2014 Elsevier Inc. All rights reserved.

SURGICAL TECHNIQUE
Components of the Telerobotic Surgical System

The robotic system consists of a master remote console, a computer controller, and a manipulator with fixed remote center kinematics connected by electrical cables and optic fibers. The master console is connected to the surgical manipulator with the camera arm and three instrumental arms. The surgeon manipulates two master handles and the movements are transmitted to the tips of the instruments by the highly sensitive motion trigger sensor. The surgical arm cart provides three degrees of freedom (pitch, yaw, insertion), and the tip of the instrument is characterized by a mechanical cable-driven wrist (EndoWrist), providing four more degrees of freedom (internal pitch, internal yaw, rotation, and grip).

This system overcomes many of the technical obstacles found in traditional thoracoscopic surgery.

- The robotic system provides stereoscopic binocular vision allowing the surgeon depth perception and high optical resolution. Three-dimensional imaging is one of the advantages over traditional VATS images, which are two-dimensionally displayed in the monitor.
- A stable camera platform is another great benefit of the robotic system. The scope is held by the central arm and is directly controlled by the surgeon at the console, permitting an increased close vision for fine dissection and panoramic vision of the whole thoracic cavity. In addition, the robotic camera holder liberates the bedside assistant's hands, allowing him or her to perform other functions.
- Magnified video imaging up to 10 times the actual size is helpful to delineate anatomic relationships and is ideal for narrow spaces, such as the anterior mediastinum or pelvis.
- Robotic instruments reproduce the human hand's degrees of freedom, which are lost during VATS surgery. This greatly enhances the surgeon's ability to manipulate the hilar structures and lobar vessels. Three degrees of freedom are conferred by the robotic arm, which allows pitch, yaw, and insertion movements. Four degrees are conferred by the mechanical wrist located inside the chest cavity (internal pitch, internal yaw, rotation, and grip).
- Downscaling of surgeon movements: the robotic system is a transducer of the surgeon's movements in more fine ones of the instrument's tips.

- Indexing is another advantage of robotic systems over traditional VATS instruments.
- Tremor filter: robotic system software is able to filter (6 Hz) surgeon hand tremors by a transducer that reproduces only the desired movements in the operative field.

Preoperative and Patient Positioning

General anesthesia with double-lumen intubation is mandatory. The patient is positioned in a lateral decubitus position, such as for a posterolateral thoracotomy, with the operating table flexed at the scapula tip level. In case of female patients, a pillow can be positioned under the hip to have patient's hip and scapula level on the same line (**Fig. 1**).

The appropriate sites of the incisions are essential for the success of the procedure, and to avoid any arm impingement during the operation. For this reason a minimum distance of 6 to 8 cm from each arm is required (**Fig. 2**). Generally, the first port is placed in the seventh to eighth intercostal space on the postirior axillary line. In this site the camera (30-degree angled down scope) is positioned. Then, an exploration of the chest cavity is performed by the camera to provide important information that could alter the programed procedure. Next, the other port incisions (8 mm) can be performed:

1) 6th–7th intercostal space at distance of 6 cm postirior to the camera port (when possible is preferibly to follow the e same intercostal space)
2) 4th–5th intercostal space (anterior axillary line)
3) auscultatory area

However, the port placement varies, and the best port positioning is assessed during the exploration of chest cavity, in relation to the fissure and to the shape of each patient's thorax. A utility port

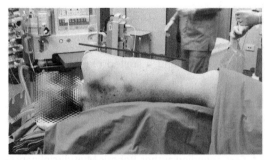

Fig. 1. Position of the patient: as with a posterolateral thoracotomy, with the operating table flexed at the scapula tip level. The hip and the scapula must be on the same line (*red line*).

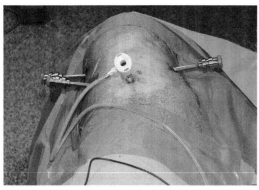

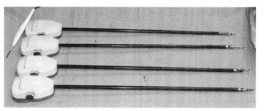

Fig. 3. Robotic instrumentation: Cadiere forceps, permanent cautery hook (monopolar cautery), fenestrated forceps (bipolar cautery), prograsp forceps.

Fig. 2. The camera port (12 mm) is placed into the seventh to eighth intercostal space on the midaxillary line. The other ports are performed in the sixth to seventh intercostal space on the posterior axillary line, in the fourth to fifth intercostal space on the anterior axillary line, and in the ausculatory area (for the fourth arm).

between the camera port and the anterior robotic port can be positioned for the assistant surgeon, who has to introduce stapler or suction. The incision in the anterior axillary line may be enlarged to 3 cm as utility incision. However, with an appropriate learning curve, a totally endoscopic procedure can be performed without the utility incision.

Once performed the port incisions, the surgical cart can be positioned from the head of the patient. The center of the column of the surgical cart must be in line with the camera port and the longitudinal axis of the patient. This fact is mandatory to avoid impingement of the robotic arms. The layout is the same for the right and left side.

Robotic Dissection

The hilum dissection is performed using a Cadiere forceps and Hook (monopolar) or Maryland (bipolar). The Cadiere forceps can be used through the fourth arm for lung retraction to obtain the optimal exposure of the mediastinum. The dissection of each hilar structure is performed by electrocautery (Hook) and a blunt instrument (Cadiere) (**Figs. 3** and **4**). Then, when the structures are sufficiently mobilized a sling is passed to facilitate the stapler positioning. However, small arteries can be safely ligated with a double tie of linen 2.5 and a clip (Hem-o-lok, WECK; TFX Medical Ltd, High Wycomb, UK) can be precisely applied by the surgeon on resected specimen. Recently, a new robotic instrument is available for vessel section: Vessel Sealer can be used on vessels smaller than 7 mm. The vein is safely resected by mechanical stapler. The bronchus step is generally performed after the vascular ones. It consists of

sweeping tissue along the lobar bronchus so that lobar bronchial nodes can be completely removed with the specimen. After the isolation and passing a sling, the resection of the bronchus is performed with a staple. The bronchial stump is then tested under water for air leaks. When possible, the completion of the fissure is performed at the end of the procedure, before removal of the specimen. Finally, the specimen is placed in a sterile plastic bag and removed through the anterior port, which is enlarged without rib spearing.

With regards to the adequacy of lymphadenectomy, there are no limitations in lymph node dissection. All the accessible nodal stations are systematically removed to ensure proper staging of the lung cancer. Lymph node dissection is performed with a Cadiere and a Hook, both during the dissection (N9, N10, N11) and at the end of the operation, when mediastinal stations (N2, N3, N4, N5-6 for left side, N7, N8) are easier to reach. Currently, the lymph node samplings are made from stations that are more likely involved in tumors originating from a particular lobe, according to Naruke classification[11]: right upper lobe (prevascular and retrotracheal N3, upper and lower paratracheal N2-4R, N7), middle lobe (N3 and subcarinal N7), right lower lobe (N7, N8, N9), left upper lobe (subaortic N5 and para-aortic N6), and left lower lobe (N7, N8, N9).

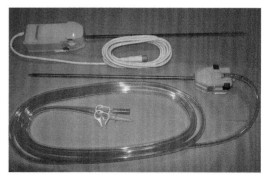

Fig. 4. The recent robotic instrumentation: vessel sealer and robotic irrigator.

STEPS FOR SPECIFIC ANATOMIC RESECTIONS

Video robotic lobectomy follows the standard surgical steps of open thoracic surgery. However, priorities are not strictly set.

Right Upper Lobectomy

The upper lobe vein is cleaned, isolated, and surrounded with a sling. From the posterior side, the bronchus is cleaned and surrounded by a sling. Then, the lobe is retracted forward to expose the pulmonary artery and the truncus anterior branch, which is identified and encircled with a sling. The dissection of the pulmonary parenchyma at confluence between the major and minor fissure permits identification of the ascending branch or branches. The small ascending vessel is generally double tied (linen 2.5). When everything is ready, the vein is divided by a stapler, then the artery, and finally the bronchus. The minor fissure is generally the last structure to be controlled.

Middle Lobectomy

The dissection of the pulmonary parenchyma at the confluence between the major and minor fissure permits identification of the arterial branch. However, the horizontal fissure is generally incomplete; thus, an anterior exposure of the mediastinum permits exposure of the upper pulmonary vein and its middle lobe branch. The second step is to deal with the bronchus, which is resected using a stapler. This allows exposure of the artery branch, which can be divided by double tie (generally) or stapler. The minor fissure is generally the last structure to be controlled.

Right Lower Lobectomy

The pulmonary ligament is incised and the pulmonary vein cleaned and surrounded by a sling. The dissection of the pulmonary parenchyma at the confluence between the major and minor fissure permits identification the superior segment branch and the basal artery, which are divided by ligation or stapler. The lower lobe is retracted inferiorly, and the major fissure can be controlled by stapler. Finally, the lower bronchus is divided with care taken to preserve the middle lobe bronchus.

Left Upper Lobectomy

The lingular branches are firstly divided (generally with double ligation), after dissection of the pulmonary parenchyma in the fissure. The dissection continues upward to identify the posterior arterial branches, which originates in the fissure along the inner curve of the pulmonary artery. These branches can be divided by ligation or stapler,

according to the size of the vessel. Often, the truncus anterior artery is covered by the upper bronchus. In this phase the fourth arm is very useful because it allows one to obtain the right tension and to safely control the truncus anterior, so that it can be divided by ligation or stapler (generally). The dissection proceeds on the anterior mediastinum to identify the superior vein that is divided by stapler. The bronchus can be cleared and resected.

Left Lower Lobectomy

The pulmonary ligament is incised and the pulmonary vein identified and cleared. The dissection of the pulmonary parenchyma in the fissure permits identification the superior segment branch and the basal segmental branch, which are generally divided by ligation or stapler, respectively. The fissure now can be safely controlled by stapler, anteriorly and posteriorly. The bronchus is the last element: it is cleaned from the surrounding tissue and divided by stapler.

PERSONAL EXPERIENCE

Since February 2001, more than 400 patients were selected for robotic procedures, ranging from simple operations, such as benign tumor excision, to complex ones, such as major lung resections. A total of 235 patients underwent robotic lobectomy (158 men, 77 women; mean age 63.6 years, range 30–85). Preoperative assessment included chest radiograph, bronchoscopy, blood tumor markers, chest and upper abdomen computed tomography scan, and positron emission tomography scan. Mediastinoscopy was not performed in those cases with no lymph node enlargement at computed tomography scan and/or of negative lymph node at positron emission tomography scan. Patients were found to have clinical stage I NSCLC disease. Operative mean time was 215 minutes (range, 110–380), including docking time. There were 15 (6.4%) conversions to open thoracotomy caused by bleeding from pulmonary vein (two), pleural adhesion (five), or fused fissure (eight). These last cases occurred at the very beginning of our series. Now, with gained experience, the absence of fissure is not a criteria for conversion. From September 2010, we use a totally endoscopic technique, but in two cases a service entrance (3 cm, without rib sparing) was performed because of hilar calcified lymph nodes, which made the totally endoscopic dissection of the artery branches unsafe (one case, right upper lobectomy), and because of unexpected tumor invasion of the vein, which required its intrapericarial isolation (one case, left upper lobectomy). However, both procedures were successfully completed. Chest tube mean duration was 2.1 days (range, 2–28). The oncologic outcomes of the first 120 were published in a recent multi-institutional study, obtaining a global actuarial 5-year survival of 80%, with a mean follow-up period of 27 months. With regard to the other 109 patients, the actuarial 5-year overall survival was 79%, with a mean follow-up of 17 months.

COMMENT

Originally, robotic systems were developed for cardiac surgery: the first internal mammary artery grafting was performed in 1999 and then in 2000.[12,13] After these experiences, robotic systems were applied in other fields, such as thoracic surgery, with a large range of procedures, starting from simple ones like the resection of anterior or posterior mediastinal masses.[14–16] However, robotic technology has added certain advantages especially in minimally invasive anatomic lung resection. In 2002 we reported the encouraging results of five pulmonary lobectomies performed with the aid of robotic technology.[17] Then, we and other authors described the use of robotic systems to perform lower lobectomy for stage I NSCLC.[18–20] These first experiences demonstrated the safety and feasibility of robotic lobectomy for early stage lung cancer. However, they were associated with increased operative time in respect to conventional surgery. This was partly related to the necessity of adequate surgical training for acquiring new skills[21] and to the instrumentation initially available, which was designed to use on coronary vessels and was often inadequate for thoracic surgery. In addition, during the first period of clinical use of the robotic system, there was no standardized technique. Gharagozloo and coworkers[22] described a hybrid technique: the robotic arms are positioned at the eighth (camera), sixth, and fifth intercostal space for the dissection of hilar structures. After the dissection phase, the robot is removed, and the surgeon returns to the operating table for vascular, bronchial, and parenchymal division. Ninan and Dylewski[23] described a robotic lobectomy with three arms: the robotic camera port is placed in the fifth or sixth intercostal space, directly over the midfissure area. The two other ports are placed in the same intercostal space anteriorly and posteriorly, to avoid multiple intercostal neurovascular bundles. A utility port was inserted over the eleventh rib and bluntly tunneled over the ninth rib, entering in the chest cavity through the eighth intercostal space.[23] Cerfolio and

coworkers[24] described robotic lobectomy with four robotic arms all positioned along seventh rib, between the midaxillary line and the paravertebral line, at a minimum distance of 9 cm from each other.

Nevertheless, advanced training on robotic systems and dedicated instruments allowed the improvement of robotic application for lung lobectomy on large series. Some authors reported the use of robotic system on large cohort for lobectomy[22–27] and for segmentectomy[28] with low conversion rate and low morbidity and mortality, demonstrating its feasibility and safety (**Table 1**).

Some claimed benefits arose from these studies on robotic lobectomy. First, the three-dimensional high-definition view with depth perception is a remarkable improvement over the conventional thoracoscopic views, which display a two-dimensional image on the monitor. In addition, magnification allows precise imaging of restricted areas and a panoramic view of the operative field. Second, robotic instruments (seven degrees of freedom, which were lost during the VATS surgery) reproduce the human-wrist movement inside the chest cavity, and the fulcrum effect of thoracoscopic instruments is avoided. These features greatly enhance the surgeon's ability to manipulate the hilar structure and lobar vessels. In a recent paper by Schimd and colleagues[29] a hybrid VATS-robotic minimally invasive sleeve lobectomy was reported without intraoperative complications. This study underlined how the articulation of robotic instruments is very useful for suturing and performing anastomosis, also in remote anatomic areas. This reinforces the assumption that the robot offers a benefit mainly in very complex procedures.

However, an important criticism is represented by the oncologic results. The first key point regards lymph node dissection: some recent studies comparing mediastinal lymph node dissection have demonstrated equivalence between robotic and open approaches, both for total number of resected lymph node and the median number of N1 and N2 lymph node stations assessed.[24,28] In addition, it should be recognized that robotics, thanks to its three dimensional vision and to the articulation of the instruments, allowed greater confidence in dissecting N1 lymph nodes adjacent to the lobar arteries and bronchus. This may ultimately have an impact on oncologic outcomes in the long term, but in the immediacy of the operation it permits easier and safer passage of the stapler.

The second key point is represented by the long-term outcomes. The only study on a large cohort evaluating robotic lobectomy in terms

Table 1
Summary of perioperative outcomes for patients who underwent robotic video-assisted thoracic surgery (lobectomy/segmentectomy)

	Number of Patients	Operative Time (min)	Lymph Node Resected	Conversion Rate (%)	Complication Rate (%)	Mortality Rate (%)	Postoperative Stay (d)
Augustin et al	26	228	NR	19.2	15.4	0	11 (7–53)
Ninam et al	74	150	5	2.6	12.2	0	3
Varonesi et al	54	260	15 (4–7)	13.0	20.4	0	6 (4–24)
Gharagozloo et al	100	216	12 ± 3	1.0	21.0	3.0	4 (3–42)
Park et al	34	218	4 (2–7)	11.8	26.5	0	2–14
Cerfolio et al	118	134	17	10.1	27	0	2 (1–7)
Our experience	235	215	NR	6.4	17	0.4	4.4

Abbreviation: NR, Not Reported.

of long-term survival is the one by Park and colleagues.[30] They obtained a 5-year overall survival of 80% with a median follow-up of 27 months; it increases to 91% and 88% if stage IA and IB, respectively, were considered.

Another important criticism is represented by the cost of a robotic system. Park and Flores[31] conducted the only cost analysis to date, comparing conventional VATS,[31] robotic approaches, and open thoracotomy in a retrospective study. They concluded that robotic VATS was more expensive than conventional VATS, but cheaper than open thoracotomy. The main factor in reducing the costs of VATS and robotic VATS compared with thoracotomy was the reduced length of hospitalization.[31]

In conclusion, robotic lobectomy should not be considered experimental, but an accepted minimally invasive thoracic surgical technique. Future evaluation of differences among robotic, VATS, and thoracotomy approaches to thoracic diseases is warranted in terms of long-term outcomes.

REFERENCES

1. Lung Cancer Study Group, Ginsberg RJ, Rubinstein LV. Randomised trial of lobectomy versus limited resection for T1N0 non-small cell lung cancer. Ann Thorac Surg 1995;60:615–23.
2. Lewis RJ, Caccavale RJ, Bocage JP, et al. Video assisted thoracic surgical non-rib spearing simultaneously stapled lobectomy. Chest 1999;116:1119–24.
3. Demmy TL, Curtis JJ. Minimally-invasive lobectomy directed toward frail and high-risk patients: a case control study. Ann Thorac Surg 1999;68:194–200.
4. McKenna RJ, Houck W, Fuller CB. Video assisted thoracic surgery lobectomy: experience with 1,100 cases. Ann Thorac Surg 2006;81:421–6.
5. Daniels LJ, Balderson SS, Onaitis MW, et al. Thoracoscopic lobectomy: a safe and effective strategy for patients with stage I lung cancer. Ann Thorac Surg 2002;74:860–4.
6. Nagahiro I, Andou A, Aoe M, et al. Pulmonary function, postoperative pain, and serum cytokine level after lobectomy: a comparison of VATS and conventional procedure. Ann Thorac Surg 2001;72:362–5.
7. Miller DL, Allen MS. Set-up and present indications: video-assisted thoracic surgery. Semin Thorac Cardiovasc Surg 1993;5(4):280–3.
8. Osmote K, Feussner H, Ungeheurer A, et al. Self guided camera control. Am J Surg 1999;177:321–4.
9. Vassiliades TA Jr, Nielsen JL. Alternative approaches in off-pump redo coronary artery bypass grafting. Heart Surg Forum 2000;3:203–6.
10. Stephenson ER, Sankholkar S, Ducko CT, et al. Robotically assisted microsurgery for endoscopic coronary artery bypass grafting. Ann Thorac Surg 1998;66:1064–7.
11. Naruke T, Suemasu K, Ishikawa S. Lymph node mapping and curability of various levels of metastases in resected lung cancer. J Thorac Cardiovasc Surg 1978;76:832.
12. Carpentier A, Louimel D, Aupacie B, et al. Computer-assisted cardiac surgery. Lancet 1999;353:379–80.
13. Kappert U, Ciehon R, Guliemos V, et al. Robotic-enhanced Dresden technique for minimally invasive bilateral mammary artery grafining. Heart Surg Forum 2000;3:319–21.
14. Yoshino I, Hashizume M, Shimada M, et al. Thoracoscopic thymomectomy with the da Vinci computer-

enhanced surgical system. J Thorac Cardiovasc Surg 2001;122(4):783–5.

15. Bodner J, Wykypiel H, Greiner A, et al. Early experience with robot-assisted surgery for mediastinal masses. Ann Thorac Surg 2004;78(1):259–65 [discussion: 265–6].

16. Rea F, Marulli G, Bortolotti L, et al. Experience with the "da Vinci" robotic system for thymectomy in patients with myasthenia gravis: report of 33 cases. Ann Thorac Surg 2006;81(2):455–9.

17. Melfi FM, Menconi GF, Mariani AM, et al. Early experience with robotic technology for thoracoscopic surgery. Eur J Cardiothorac Surg 2002;21(5):864–8.

18. Ashton RC Jr, Connery CP, Swistel DG, et al. Robot-assisted lobectomy. J Thorac Cardiovasc Surg 2003;126(1):292–3.

19. Bodner J, Wykypiel H, Wetscher G, et al. First experiences with the da Vinci operating robot in thoracic surgery. Eur J Cardiothorac Surg 2004;25(5):844–51.

20. Melfi FM, Ambrogi MC, Mussi A, et al. Video robotic lobectomy. Multimed Man Cardiothorac Surg 2005; 2005(628). mmcts.2004.000448.

21. Meyer M, Gharagozloo F, Tempesta B, et al. The learning curve of robotic lobectomy. Int J Med Robot 2012;8(4):448–52.

22. Gharagozloo F, Margolis M, Tempesta B, et al. Robot-assisted lobectomy for early-stage lung cancer: report of 100 consecutive cases. Ann Thorac Surg 2009;88:380–4.

23. Ninan M, Dylewski MR. Total port-access robot-assisted pulmonary lobectomy without utility thoracotomy. Eur J Cardiothorac Surg 2010;38:231–2.

24. Cerfolio RJ, Bryant BS, Skylizard L, et al. Initial consecutive experience of completely portal robotic pulmonary resection with 4 arms. J Thorac Cardiovasc Surg 2011;142:740–6.

25. Park BJ, Flores RM, Rusch VW. Robotic assistance for video-assisted thoracic surgical lobectomy: technique and initial results. J Thorac Cardiovasc Surg 2006;131(1):54–9.

26. Augustin F, Bodner J, Wykypiel H, et al. Initial experience with robotic lung lobectomy: report of two different approaches. Surg Endosc 2011;25: 108–13.

27. Pardolesi A, Park B, Petrella F, et al. Robotic anatomic segmentectomy of the lung: technical aspects and initial results. Ann Thorac Surg 2012; 94(3):929–34.

28. Veronesi G, Galetta D, Maisonneuve P, et al. Four-arm robotic lobectomy for the treatment of early-stage lung cancer. J Thorac Cardiovasc Surg 2010;140:19–25.

29. Schmid T, Augustin F, Kainz G, et al. Hybrid video-assisted thoracic surgery-robotic minimally invasive right upper lobe sleeve lobectomy. Ann Thorac Surg 2011;91(6):1961–5.

30. Park BJ, Melfi F, Mussi A, et al. Robotic lobectomy for non–small cell lung cancer (NSCLC): long-term oncologic results. J Thorac Cardiovasc Surg 2012; 143:383–9.

31. Park BJ, Flores RM. Cost comparison of robotic, video-assisted thoracic surgery and thoracotomy approaches to pulmonary lobectomy. Thorac Surg Clin 2008;18:297–300, vii.

Total Port Approach for Robotic Lobectomy

Robert J. Cerfolio, MD, MBA

KEYWORDS

• Lobectomy • Robotic lobectomy • Thoracic surgery • Lung cancer • Lymph node dissection

KEY POINTS

- The current literature shows that robotic surgery is safe and efficient and has similar survival rates compared with the open and video-assisted thoracoscopic surgery (VATS) approaches.
- The surgeon can provide an R0 resection in patients with cancer; even those with large tumors (up to 10 cm).
- Outstanding mediastinal and hilar lymph node resections are achievable.
- Technical modifications lead to decreased operative times and may improve the ability to teach as well as decreasing patient morbidity and surgeon frustration during the learning process.
- Although hospitals are acquiring more robots for other specialties besides thoracic surgery, the capital cost, service contract costs, and equipment costs have to be carefully considered and studied.
- Patient selection is critical, especially during the learning process.
- In our opinion, there are few, if any, achievable benefits of using a robotic system compared with VATS when performing a sympathotomy for patients with hyperhidrosis or a pulmonary wedge resection for tissue diagnosis for patients with interstitial lung disease.
- Although further studies are needed, there has been an expansion of interest in robotics in general thoracic surgery and longer survival studies are needed.

Robotic surgery is not only becoming the standard of care in urology and gynecology but it is also gaining momentum in thoracic surgery. Some types of minimally invasive surgery (MIS) such as video-assisted thoracoscopic surgery (VATS) are limited by two-dimensional visualization, a camera that often requires cleaning, nonwristed instruments, and ergonomic discomfort. Because minimally invasive platforms have now been shown to improve outcomes from lung resection,[1,2] patient and surgeon alike have accepted MIS. Robotics is an MIS platform that offers distinct advantages compared with VATS and has led to the growth of robotic surgery. Robotic pulmonary resection may also lead to improved lymph node dissection, less blood loss, and improved

resection of hilar (N1) lymph nodes off the pulmonary artery.[3–7] It also has been purported to cause less pain then VATS.[8] However, robotic surgery has limitations, which include a longer setup time (more trocars and ports are used and docking time is required), higher initial capital costs, lack of ability to palpate the lung or have haptic feedback, and it requires more specialized equipment.

Enthusiasm for robots has stemmed from the success in mediastinal resections and esophageal resections. Although this article is limited to pulmonary resections, robots have been successful in the mediastinum and esophagus for both malignant and benign esophageal lesions, so thoracic surgeons have extended the use of the robot for pulmonary resection.

Disclosure: Proctor for Intuitive.
Lung Cancer Research, 739 Zeigler Research Building, 703 19th Street South, Birmingham, AL 35294-0007, USA
E-mail address: rcerfolio@uabmc.edu

Thorac Surg Clin 24 (2014) 151–156
http://dx.doi.org/10.1016/j.thorsurg.2014.02.006
1547-4127/14/$ – see front matter © 2014 Elsevier Inc. All rights reserved.

An international writing committee has suggested nomenclature for robotic pulmonary resection (**Table 1**). In this article (not yet published), completely portal is abbreviated as CPRL-4 and robotic assisted is abbreviated as RATS. This nomenclature differentiates the different ways of performing robotic pulmonary resection. The important point is that the robot has now been used on more than 1000 patients to safely perform pulmonary resections and provides a minimally invasive surgical method.

On comparing CPRL-4 with RATS, CPRL-4 offers a completely closed environment; less third spacing, introducing warm humidified CO_2; and more working room. But, CRPL-4 does not allow palpation of the lung.

OPERATIVE METHODS

There are several different techniques used to perform the operation. Veronesi and Melfi[9] in 2011 reported the safety of a 4-arm robot-assisted (not completely portal) lobectomy (using a access incision of 3–4 cm as used by VATS surgeons). Ninan and Dylewski[3] in 2010 reported the effectiveness of a completely portal robotic lobectomy using 3 arms (CPRL-3) in 74 patients. Gharagozloo and colleagues[7] in 2009 reported outcomes using a hybrid technique.[1] **Fig. 1B** shows the procedure.

We prefer the CPRL-4 method. As shown in **Fig. 2**, the pleural space is entered over the top of the seventh rib using a 5-mm port in the midaxillary line or as anteriorly as possible and guided by a 5-mm scope. A 5-mm VATS camera is used to ensure entry into the pleural space and warmed CO_2 is insufflated to drive the diaphragm inferiorly. This incision is eventually enlarged to allow a 12-mm port and it serves as robotic arm 1 (for right-sided operations). A paravertebral block is performed posteriorly using a local anesthetic and a 21-gauge needle from ribs 3 to 11. The needle is used to help select the ideal location for the second incision, which is the most posterior incision. The location chosen is 2 ribs below the major fissure and as far posterior in the chest as possible, just anterior to the spinal processes of the vertebral body. A 5-mm incision is made and a 5-mm reusable metal da Vinci trocar is placed. This is the position for robotic arm 3. The next few incisions are carefully planned and marked on the skin before making them. Ten centimeters anterior to the most posterior incision and along the same rib (most commonly rib 8) a third incision is planned. It is an incision for an 8-mm port and its trocar is an 8-mm metal reusable da Vinci trocar, which is docked with robotic arm 2. A fourth incision is marked on the skin and again planned but not made 9 cm anteriorly to this port, along the same rib as shown in **Fig. 2**. This mark will eventually be used for the robotic camera. A 12-mm plastic disposable port is used for the 12-mm camera and, if the 8-mm camera is used, an 8-mm metal reusable trocar is placed. Before making these 2 incisions a 21-gauge needle is used to identify the most anteriorly inferior aspect of the chest

Table 1
Operative characteristics for the proposed nomenclature system for general thoracic robotic operations

	Completely Portal Robotic	Robotic Assisted
Abbreviation suggested	Yes - CPRL	Yes - RAL
Designation uses the number of robotic arms used	Yes	Yes
Example provided for lobectomy using 4 arms	CPRL - 4	RAL - 4
Example provided for thymectomy using 3 arms	CPT - 3	RAT - 3
Rib spreading	No	No
Access or utility incision made	No	Yes
CO_2 insufflation used	Yes	Sometimes
Communication between pleural space air and ambient air in operating room	No	Yes
Trocars placed through all incisions	Yes	No
Incisions bigger than the trocars used	No	Yes
Site of specimen removal	Usually over anterior aspect of 10th rib	Usually over anterior aspect of fourth rib

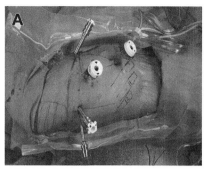
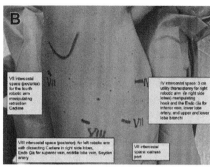

Fig. 1. (*A*) Intraoperative view of port placement for a CPRL-4 in the right chest. The patient's head is at the left of the picture, and the feet are at the right. The anterior chest is at the top and the back is at the bottom. The scapula is outlined. (*B*) Intraoperative view of port placement and utility incision for a robotic assisted lobectomy in the right chest using 3 arms. The patient's head is at the top of the picture and the anterior chest is to the right of the picture.

that is just above the diaphragmatic fibers. This incision has a 15-mm port and serves as the access port. A plastic disposable trocar is used. No robotic arms are attached to the trocar that is placed in this incision. This incision is carefully planned. It is made just above the diaphragm as anterior and inferior as possible in order to be between the ports used for robotic arm 1 and the camera. The access port can alternatively be

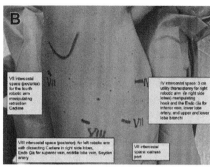

Fig. 2. The CPRL-4 technique developed in this study. It features entering the pleural space using a 5-mm port anteriorly in the midaxillary line (MAL) over the top of the seventh rib and then using a 5-mm VATS camera to make all the other incisions based on internal anatomy. The circled numbers represent the robotic arms used. C is for the camera port, A is for the 15-mm access port (which can also be placed between the camera and robotic arm 2 if space is not adequate more anteriorly). Note that robotic arm 3 is a 5-mm port, robotic arm 2 is an 8-mm port, the camera can be an 8-mm or 12-mm port depending on the camera used, and robotic arm 1 is a 12-mm port. The area with the dashed lines is the area where no incisions are made, and this is the most posterior third of the area between the midspine and the posterior edge of the scapula.

placed more posteriorly if anatomy dictates; between the camera and robotic arm 2. It should be 2 or 3 ribs lower than these two ports. This position affords room for the bedside assistant to work. Once these incisions are carefully planned and their location is confirmed, they are made and the appropriate trocars are placed. In addition, the initial 5-mm anterior port that was made first and used to introduce the VATS camera to identify the internal landmarks is then dilated to a 12-mm double cannulated port for robotic arm 1. The robot is driven over the patient's shoulder on a 15° angle and attached to the 4 ports. In general, only 4 robotic instruments are used for all of these operations: the Cadierre grasper, a 5-mm bowel grasper (used exclusively through the most posterior port that is attached to robotic arm 3, which serves as a retractor of the lung), the Maryland forceps, and a cautery spatula. See **Fig. 1**A for interoperative views.

RESULTS

Recent literature shows that robotic pulmonary resection is safe and oncologically sound by allowing R0 resection with excellent lymph node removal.[3,4,8,10]

Our series reports on 168 patients who underwent robotic resection for non–small cell lung cancer (NSCLC) and were matched (3:1) with patients who had a pulmonary resection via nerve-sparing and rib-sparing thoracotomy. There was no statistically significant difference in the total number of lymph nodes removed or in the median number of N2 or N1 lymph node stations assessed. In addition, there was significantly less blood loss (35 vs 90 mL, $P = .03$), shorter chest tube duration (1.5 vs 3.0 days, $P<.001$), shorter hospital length of stay (2 vs 4 days, $P = .02$), lower incidence of morbidity

(27% vs 38%, $P = .05$), and lower 3-week postoperative pain score (2.5 vs 4.4, $P = .04$) favoring the CPRL-4 group. Postoperative morbidity rates were similar between the two groups. Results of CPRL-4 after technical modifications show a trend in reduction of median operative times as shown in **Fig. 3** and reduction in conversion rates (12 of the first 62 [19%] operations and 1 in the last 106 [1%], $P<.001$). The significant technical changes made were adding the fourth robotic arm posteriorly and using a 5-mm port so the surgeon can retract the lung personally; placing a vessel loop around the artery, vein, bronchus, and fissures to help guide the stapler; the removal of the tumor above the diaphragm; and using CO_2 insufflation.

A recent publication by Park and colleagues[4] (2012) that evaluated 325 patients who underwent robotic lobectomy for early stage NSCLC also showed minimal morbidity and mortality. Survival rates were similar to those for similar staged patients who underwent lobectomy by VATS or thoracotomy.

DISCUSSION

The advantages of the robot compared with VATS include improved visualization, improved instrumentation that provides the surgeon with more degrees of movement, better lymph node visualization and dissection, high magnification, the ability to teach using a dual console, and the simulator. However, the disadvantages include limited platform availability as well as the capital and maintenance costs and expensive software required for the robot.[8] An additional drawback is that instruments have to be replaced after 10 to 20 uses based on whether they are 5 or 8 mm respectively. In addition, a complete portal approach does not allow the surgeon to palpate the lung.

The reasons to perform MIS include the immunologic benefits of a minimally invasive, non–rib-spreading operation that may lead to improved survival for patients with NSCLC.[2,5,11,12] The adoption of the robot for pulmonary resection will depend on several factors: the availability of the robotic platform to the thoracic surgeon; the cost of the operation; the measured and perceived benefits to the patient, hospital, and surgeon; and the time it takes to perform the operation. Most important is the surgeon's current enthusiasm for the VATS lobectomy to be performed: MIS is the method of the future. If a team is already adept at VATS lobectomy and thinks that the lymph node dissection is adequate, the desire to adopt robotic pulmonary resection into the practice will be low. However, if the lymph node dissection during VATS lobectomy was, as in our experience, suboptimal and difficult to teach, then it will probably be high.

Many general thoracic surgeons are eager to learn robotic surgical systems and many centers are starting to use them. This eagerness must be tempered with proper training, careful patient selection, and intelligent program building. The credentialing of robotic proficiency needs to be systemically promulgated. At present, the decision regarding credentialing is made on an institutional level. Although the literature now contains articles that show the technical and oncologic safety of robotic pulmonary resection and robotic thymectomy, proper training of the team is critical to maintain patient safety.

We think that the proper sequence of training leads to a program's success. There are many lessons that we learned but that cannot be ascribed a P value and cannot be assessed using

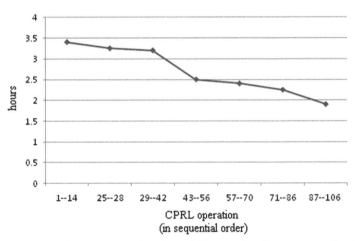

Fig. 3. Median operative times (skin incision to skin closure) for completed CPRL-4 over time in sequential order.

Table 2
Lessons learned: common problems and modifications and solutions

Problem	Modification
Robotic arms hitting	Make each port at least 8-cm to 9-cm apart, use arm 3 for the posterior port, dock using camera sweet spot
Cannot take down inferior pulmonary ligament without repositioning camera	Place robotic camera port no higher than the eighth intercostal space
Exposures are difficult, reliant on bedside assistant (via 15-mm port) who is different for each case	Use robotic arm 3 as the posterior port and use it to retract the lung using a 5-mm bowel grasper
Stapling the fissure is more difficult than open	Ensure surgeon's view on console is set to wide, pull camera back into trocar for more panoramic view
Small bleeding prevents visualization and suction removes CO_2 and decreases visibility	Remove blood using rolled-up sponges; activate sucker only when submerged under blood, use fenestrated bipolar instrument for hemostasis
One surgeon operates while the other watches	The attending surgeon can assist and proctor the resident using robotic arm 3, while the resident uses arms 1 and 2 to dissect, if dual consoles are available
Vessel stapling is performed by the assistant and is dangerous	Test the ideal port to introduce the vascular stapler, using the straight robotic arms as a guide (use a vessel loop to guide stapler placement) awaiting robotic stapler
Costs are high	Minimize costs by using reusable metal instead of plastic ports, only 3 to 4 robotic instruments are needed per operation, clip small PA branches instead of using a stapler
Takes too long	Surgeon remains at the console, trusts bedside assistant to fire the stapler on vessel, do more cases in short period of time, have dedicated team
Most posterior port can bleed	Use an 5-mm metal port posteriorly; make it anterior to a point two-thirds between the posterior scapular edge and the spine
Room between anterior port and camera too close for assistant to work comfortably	Carefully plan the incisions to maximize the triangle formed by the anterior port, the camera port, and the 15-mm working port; initially select patients taller than 152 cm with a BMI <35 kg/m^2. Use a 0° camera instead of a 30 down
Blood dripping onto operative field from camera port	Replace camera port with a balloon-inflatable port
Camera hitting hip	Clutch camera port, switch to 30 up or 0° lens
Lots of adhesions	Start by taking these down with VATS and place robot camera in a 15-mm access incision
Arms not working as surgeon is operating	Ensure the trocar is in the chest, ensure blue light is on, ensure the robot is fastened to the port, ensure hands not maxed at console (ie, clutch) finally look at robot arms at patient and fix pitch/yaw limits of robot
15-mm access port too small for specimen extraction	Deliver bag strings through access incision; undock robot; open bag but avoid spillage; enlarge incision, then, working inside the bag, reach into bag with lung clamp and deliver side part of the lobe first, then pull rest of lobe slowly out, working inside the bag, then remove bag with lobe

Abbreviations: BMI, body mass index; PA, pulmonary artery.

conventional scientific evidence-based methods. The points made in **Table 2** thus represent our opinion after having performed more than 900 robotic operations and after having proctored many surgeons at different centers. Some of the difficult lessons that we learned in our initial experience may be of benefit to other clinicians.[13]

In conclusion, the current literature shows that robotic surgery is safe and efficient and has similar survival rates compared with the open and VATS approaches. The surgeon can provide an R0 resection in patients with cancer, even in those with large tumors (up to 10 cm). In addition, an outstanding mediastinal and hilar lymph node resection is achievable. Technical modifications lead to decreased operative times and may improve the ability to teach as well as decreasing patient morbidity and surgeon frustration during the learning process. Even though hospitals are acquiring more robots for other specialties besides thoracic surgery, the capital cost, service contract costs, and equipment costs have to be carefully considered and studied. Patient selection is critical, especially during the learning process. In our opinion, there are few, if any, achievable benefits of using a robotic system rather than VATS when performing a sympathotomy for patients with hyperhidrosis or a pulmonary wedge resection for tissue diagnosis for patients with interstitial lung disease. Although further studies are needed, there has been an expansion of interest in robotics in general thoracic surgery and longer survival studies are needed.

REFERENCES

1. Mahtabifard A, DeArmond DT, Fuller CB, et al. Video-assisted thoracoscopic surgery for stage 1 non-small cell lung cancer. Thorac Surg Clin 2007; 17:223–31.
2. Flores RM, Ihekweasu UN, Rizk N, et al. Patterns of recurrence and incidence of second primary tumors after lobectomy by means of video-assisted thoracoscopic surgery (VATS) versus thoracotomy for lung cancer. J Thorac Cardiovasc Surg 2011;141: 59–64.
3. Ninan M, Dylewski MR. Total port-access robot assisted pulmonary lobectomy without utility thoracotomy. Eur J Cardiothorac Surg 2010;38:231–2.
4. Park BJ, Melfi F, Mussi A, et al. Robotic lobectomy for non-small cell lung cancer (NSCLC): long-term oncologic results. J Thorac Cardiovasc Surg 2012; 143:383–9.
5. Whitson BA, Groth SS, Duval SS, et al. Surgery for early stage non-small cell lung cancer: a systematic review of the video-assisted thoracoscopic surgery versus thoracotomy approach to lobectomy. Ann Thorac Surg 2008;86:2008–18.
6. Cerfolio RJ. Pulmonary resection in the 21st century the role of robotics. Tex Heart Inst J 2012;39(6):848–9.
7. Gharagozloo F, Margolis M, Tempesta B, et al. Robot-assisted lobectomy for early-stage lung cancer: report of 100 cases. Ann Thorac Surg 2009; 88:384.
8. Cerfolio RJ, Bryant AS. Perspectives on robotic pulmonary resection: it's current and future status. Thorac Surg Clin 2012;22(2):215–8. http://dx.doi.org/10.1016/j.thorsurg.2011.12.007.
9. Veronesi G, Agoglia BG, Melfi F, et al. Experience with robotic lobectomy fro lung cancer. Innovations (Phila) 2011;6(6):355–60.
10. Minnich DJ, Bryant AS, Cerfolio RJ. Thoracoscopic and robotic dissection of mediastinal lymph nodes [review]. Thorac Surg Clin 2012;22(2):215–8. http://dx.doi.org/10.1016/j.thorsurg.2011.12.007.
11. Yan TD, Black D, Bannon PG, et al. Systematic review and meta-analysis of randomized and non-randomized trials on safety and efficacy of video-assisted thoracic surgery lobectomy for early stage non-small cell lung cancer. J Clin Oncol 2009;27: 2553–62.
12. Swanson SJ, Miller DL, McKenna RJ Jr, et al. Comparing robot-assisted thoracic surgical lobectomy with conventional video-assisted thoracic surgical lobectomy and wedge resection: results from a multihospital database (premier). J Thorac Cardiovasc Surg 2014;147:929–37. http://dx.doi.org/10.1016/j.jtcvs.2013.09.046.
13. Cerfolio RJ, Bryant AS, Minnich DJ. Starting a robotic program in general thoracic surgery: why, how, and lessons learned. Ann Thorac Surg 2011;91(6): 1729–36. http://dx.doi.org/10.1016/j.athoracsur.2011.01.104 [discussion: 1736–7].

Robotic Lobectomy for Non–Small Cell Lung Cancer: Long-Term Oncologic Results

Bernard J. Park, MD, FACS

KEYWORDS

- Robotic lobectomy • Non–small cell lung cancer • Long-term oncologic results

KEY POINTS

- Robotic lobectomy is a safe, feasible, and reproducible approach for anatomic lung resection.
- The robotic approach produces long-term results for treatment of early-stage lung cancer that are consistent with other large surgical series using either video-assisted thoracic surgery (VATS) or thoracotomy.
- Lymphadenectomy may be superior, using the advantages of robotic technology over conventional VATS.

Lung cancer remains one of the deadliest cancers worldwide.[1] With aging and growth of the population combined with the persistence of cigarette smoking and the potential widespread adoption of computed tomography lung cancer screening,[2] there will be an increasing number of early-stage lung cancers appropriate for surgical resection. Minimally invasive video-assisted thoracic surgery (VATS) lobectomy has proved to be feasible and oncologically acceptable for isolated non–small cell lung cancer (NSCLC).[3–5] However, despite multiple studies showing this factor and clear benefits over thoracotomy, such as decreased length of stay and fewer postoperative complications,[5–7] decreased pain[8] and improved delivery and tolerance of adjuvant chemotherapy,[9] use of VATS lobectomy for treatment of early-stage lung cancer is not yet the standard approach.[10,11] The reasons for this are not entirely clear, but may be related to technical limitations, such as two-dimensional imaging and limited maneuverability of instrumentation.

To address the limitations of conventional thoracoscopy, a telerobotic surgical system was developed with three-dimensional, high-definition imaging, instrumentation with 7° of freedom and a master-slave surgical cart (da Vinci, Intuitive Surgical, Sunnyvale, CA). Initial series of robotic lobectomy for the treatment of early-stage lung cancer have reported perioperative results that showed that the approach is feasible and safe.[12–14] Subsequently, others have reported variations in technique and an increasing experience,[15,16] but only 1 series has evaluated long-term oncologic results in a large cohort of consecutive, treated patients.[17] In this article, the results of a large cohort of patients that underwent robotic lobectomy are reviewed, to analyze both the perioperative and long-term survival results to determine if it has an oncologically advantageous role in the surgical management of early NSCLC.

METHODS

A multicenter retrospective cohort trial was performed using prospectively collected data from the thoracic surgery divisions of 3 institutions: Memorial Sloan-Kettering Cancer Center, New York, The European Institute of Oncology, Milan, Italy, and Ospedale Cisanello, Pisa, Italy. The study

Disclosures: None.
Division of Thoracic Surgery, Hackensack University Medical Center, 30 Prospect Avenue, Suite 409, Hackensack, NJ 07601, USA
E-mail address: bpark@hackensackumc.org

Thorac Surg Clin 24 (2014) 157–162
http://dx.doi.org/10.1016/j.thorsurg.2014.02.011
1547-4127/14/$ – see front matter © 2014 Elsevier Inc. All rights reserved.

was approved by the Institutional Review Board of each institution, and a data transfer agreement was made. Eligible patients were those with biopsy-proven or suspected clinical stage I primary NSCLC with no evidence of locally advanced or extrathoracic disease based on computed tomography (CT) of the chest, whole body positron emission tomography/CT and mediastinoscopy (select cases) who subsequently underwent attempted robotic lobectomy for primary NSCLC. Patients with carcinoid tumor, small cell lung cancer, benign or metastatic lesions, and those not undergoing lobectomy were excluded. Information regarding preoperative characteristics, operative details, hospital course, pathologic findings, and postoperative follow-up were recorded prospectively and sent to 1 institution (Milan) for analysis.

Technique of Robotic Lobectomy

At each institution, the indications for robotic lobectomy were similar: lesions isolated to the hemithorax, resectable by lobectomy in patients with adequate cardiopulmonary reserve. Each surgeon performed robotic lobectomy using a technique that conformed to the Cancer and Leukemia Group B (CALGB) 39802 consensus report for VATS lobectomy: use of non–rib-spreading incisions, with the largest incision no greater than 8 cm, videoscopic guidance, and traditional hilar dissection.[18] The detailed technical aspects have been reported previously.[12–14] At 2 centers (Milan, Pisa), a 4-arm approach was used, whereas at the third center (New York), a 3-arm technique was used. At 2 centers (Pisa, New York), a utility incision was used from the outset, whereas at the third, a total port approach was used until the specimen was ready to be removed. All patients underwent systematic mediastinal lymph node dissection. Patients gave written informed consent to undergo robotic surgery, and operative times were measured from first incision to closure. Conversion was defined as use of a rib-spreading thoracotomy at any point after docking of the robot to the patient and initiation of robotic dissection. Complications were recorded prospectively and categorized by the National Cancer Institute Common Terminology Criteria for Adverse Events version 3.0 (http://ctep.cancer.gov/reporting/ctc.html) as either minor (grades 1, 2) or major (grade 3 or higher). Clinical and pathologic staging was performed using the 7th edition of the TNM classification.[19]

Surveillance and Follow-Up

At each institution, patients were followed postoperatively for lung cancer surveillance at least every 6 months for the initial 2 years, with history, physical examination, blood work, and chest CT and annually thereafter. Patients who did not return for follow-up evaluation were contacted by telephone, or their status was checked by the Social Security Death Index in the case of patients from the United States. Survival was calculated from the date of surgery to the date of death or last follow-up. Survival estimates were calculated with the Kaplan-Meier method and compared by the log-rank test. All analyses were performed with SAS statistical software version 8.2 (SAS Institute, Cary, NC).

RESULTS

From November, 2002 to May, 2010, 325 patients underwent robotic lobectomy for primary NSCLC at 3 centers. There were 123 consecutive patients from the center in New York during the study period; 82 patients from the center in Milan from November, 2006 to May, 2010; and 120 patients from the center in Pisa from January, 2004 to May, 2010. **Table 1** shows the patient characteristics. There was a

Table 1
Patient characteristics

Category	Result
Age, y, median (range)	66 (30–87)
Male gender, n (%)	204 (63)
Smoking status, n (%)	
Unknown	3 (1)
Never	50 (15)
Former/current	272 (84)
FEV_1, % predicted, median (range)	95 (34–166)
D_{LCO}, % predicted, median (range)	87 (11–196)
Primary tumor location, n (%)	
RUL	92 (28)
RML	29 (9)
RLL	71 (22)
RUL/ML	1 (0.3)
LUL	75 (23)
LLL	57 (18)
Histology, n (%)	
Adenocarcinoma	239 (73)
Squamous cell carcinoma	74 (23)
Other	12 (4)

Abbreviations: D_{LCO}, diffusing capacity of the lung for carbon monoxide; FEV_1, forced expiratory volume in the first second; LLL, left lower lobe; LUL, left upper lobe; RLL, right lower lobe; RML, right middle lobe; RUL, right upper lobe.

From Park BJ, Melfi F, Mussi A, et al. Robotic lobectomy for non-small cell lung cancer (NSCLC): long-term oncologic results. J Thorac Cardiovasc Surg 2012;143:383–9; with permission.

small preponderance of men, and 85% were former or current smokers. More than one-half of the procedures were upper lobectomies (92 right upper lobe [RUL], 75 left upper lobe [LUL]), and 1 patient underwent bilobectomy (RUL/middle lobe) for an upper lobe tumor invading across the horizontal fissure. Most cases were subtypes of adenocarcinoma (73%). Most patients were clinical stage I (247 IA, 63 IB) and had no preoperative therapy. One patient was stage IIIA (N2) based on mediastinoscopy and received induction chemotherapy. In all, 14% (45/325) of patients underwent preresection mediastinoscopy.

Table 2 details the perioperative results of the robotic series. Median operative time was 3.5 hours. There were no intraoperative deaths, and the conversion rate to thoracotomy was 8% (27/325). Three patients (0.9%) had conversion for minor bleeding that did not require intraoperative or postoperative transfusion. Overall morbidity rate was 25.2% (82/325) and was not different between centers (New York 26%, Milan 27%, Pisa 23%). Twelve patients had major complications (3.7%), including bronchopleural fistula (2), pulmonary embolism (3), acute renal insufficiency (3), hemorrhage (2), and myocardial infarction (2). Supraventricular tachycardia was the most common postoperative

complication, occurring in 37 patients (11.4%). Median chest tube duration was 3 days (range 1–23), and length of stay was 5 days (2–28). There was 1 in-hospital death in a patient who developed acute renal insufficiency followed by a pulmonary embolism and death on postoperative day 12.

Seventy-six percent (248/325) of patients were pathologic stage I (176 IA, 72 IB), and 78 (24%) patients were upstaged (see Table 2). The median tumor size was 2.2 cm (range 0.7–10.2 cm), and the median number of lymph node stations dissected was 5 (range 2–8). Fifty-six patients (18%) were upstaged to N1, and 21 patients (6%) were upstaged to N2. At a median follow-up of 27 months, 32 patients (10%) had recurred, with 25 dead of their disease. Most (72%) were distant (17 distant only, 6 locoregional + distant), and 28% (9/32) were locoregional only. Overall 5-year survival for the group was 80% (Fig. 1A); stage-specific survival is shown in Fig. 1B.

COMMENT

With the continued growth and aging of the population and the likely acceptance of low-dose chest CT screening of high-risk populations, the number and proportion of early-stage lung cancers diagnosed annually are likely to increase. Numerous reports from high-volume centers of excellence have shown that minimally invasive VATS lobectomy can be a feasible and safe alternative to thoracotomy lobectomy, with additional benefits that include shorter length of chest tube duration and hospital stay, lower rate of major complications, decreased acute postoperative pain, and enhanced recovery and tolerance of adjuvant therapy.[3–9] There are a few, but increasing, reports of robotic lobectomy using the purported benefits of three-dimensional imaging and wristed instrumentation for minimally invasive lung resection.[12–17] Previous robotic series have shown comparable perioperative results with those seen with VATS lobectomy, and this largest reported experience[17] also affirms that robotic lobectomy is feasible and safe with a short chest tube duration and length of stay, as well as low major morbidity (3.7%) and in-hospital mortality (0.3%). No catastrophic episodes of hemorrhage were encountered, and bleeding episodes were easily managed through standard minimally invasive surgery strategies.

This is the largest experience of totally robotic lobectomies reported to date, and the only one that has analyzed long-term oncologic outcomes in the treatment of early-stage lung cancer. It was a multicenter, international experience, with 1 center in the United States and 2 in Italy using similar patient selection criteria, surgical

Table 2
Perioperative results

Category	Result
Operative time, min (range)[a]	206 (110–383)
Chest tube, d (range)[a]	3 (1–23)
Length of stay, d (range)[a]	5 (2–28)
Complications, n (%)	
None	243 (75)
Minor	70 (21.5)
Major	12 (3.7)
Perioperative mortality	1 (0.3)
Pathologic stage, n (%)[b]	
IA	176 (54)
IB	72 (22)
IIA	41 (13)
IIB	15 (5)
IIIA	21 (6)
Tumor size, cm (range)[a]	2.2 (0.7–10.2)
Lymph node stations removed, n (range)[a]	5 (2–8)

[a] Median.
[b] 7th edition TNM classification.

From Park BJ, Melfi F, Mussi A, et al. Robotic lobectomy for non-small cell lung cancer (NSCLC): long-term oncologic results. J Thorac Cardiovasc Surg 2012;143:383–9; with permission.

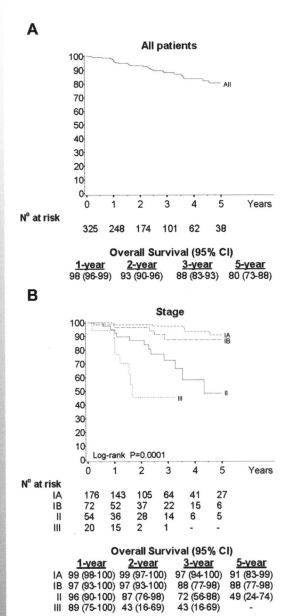

Fig. 1. (*A*) Robotic lobectomy overall survival; (*B*) stage-specific survival. CI, confidence interval. (*From* Park BJ, Melfi F, Mussi A, et al. Robotic lobectomy for non-small cell lung cancer (NSCLC): long-term oncologic results. J Thorac Cardiovasc Surg 2012;143: 383–9; with permission.)

each of the investigators performed systematic hilar and mediastinal lymph node dissection. In 2 of the centers, a 4-arm technique was used, using a fourth, small non–rib-spreading incision for placement of the fourth robotic arm for retraction, whereas a 3-arm approach was used at the third center. This minor difference in technique was likely of no clinical significance. Although most tumors were small, there were larger lesions, including a 10.2-cm tumor. Because a non–rib-spreading utility incision was used, adequate retraction was achieved easily either by robotic instrumentation alone or by the bedside assistant.

Gharagozloo and colleagues[15] described a series of 100 consecutive patients but used a hybrid VATS-robotic technique, in which the mediastinal node and initial hilar dissection were performed robotically followed by VATS for isolation and ligation of the hilar structures. Perioperative morbidity was acceptable at 21%, although in-hospital mortality was 3%. Cerfolio and colleagues[16] reported their initial experience with a 4-arm, completely portal robotic pulmonary lobectomy in 168 patients. They achieved an overall morbidity of 27% with a mean length of stay of 2.0 days and a mortality of 0%. However, neither of these series gave any detailed data with respect to pathologic stage, adjuvant therapy, or stage-specific, long-term survival.

This series[17] is the first to look at the long-term oncologic outcome of robotic lobectomy for early NSCLC. The overall and stage-specific survivals are consistent both with the largest recent series of VATS lobectomies[4,5] and the data used for the 7th edition of the lung cancer staging system, which were largely derived from conventional open surgery.[19] Onaitis and colleagues[4] reported 2-year overall survival of 80% and stage-specific survivals of 85% for stage I and 77% for stages II and higher in a cohort of 500 patients undergoing VATS lobectomy for clinical early-stage disease. Goldstraw and colleagues[19] reported 5-year overall survivals of 73% and 58% for stages IA and IB, respectively, and 46% and 36% for stages IIA and IIB. These data are consistent with that observed in this large robotic series, in which the 5-year survival for stage II patients was 49%. The very high 5-year survival for pathologic stage I patients (91% IA, 88% IB) is likely related to the fact that the median tumor size was small (2.2 cm).

One clear potential strength of the robotic approach is the thoroughness of the lymphadenectomy. In this experience of clinical stage I patients, pathologic upstaging was seen in 24% of patients with 18% N1 upstaging and 6% N2 upstaging. This finding is consistent with what would be expected in a large surgical series of lobectomy

technique, and prospective evaluation of perioperative and long-term outcome. The patient population was relatively uniform, composed of largely early-stage patients without previous treatment and with adequate cardiopulmonary reserve for lobectomy. As detailed in previous technical studies, each center used a fully robotic technique that conformed to the CALGB 39802 consensus criteria for minimally invasive lobectomy,[12–14] and

Table 3
Nodal upstaging by surgical approach

Reference	Node Status	% Upstaging VATS	% Upstaging Open	% Upstaging Robotic
Boffa[20]	N1	6.7	9.3	NR
	N2	4.9	5.0	NR
	Overall	11.6	14.3	NR
Licht et al,[21] 2013	N1	8.1	13.1	NR
	N2	3.8	11.5	NR
	Overall	11.9	24.6	NR
Park[17]	N1	NR	NR	18.0
	N2	NR	NR	6.0
	Overall	NR	NR	24.0

Abbreviation: NR, not reported.

for early-stage disease. Several recent studies analyzing the adequacy of lymphadenectomy by VATS have reported that there seems to be lower-than-expected nodal upstaging when VATS is compared with thoracotomy.[20,21] Boffa and colleagues[20] showed that N1 upstaging in 11,531 cases from the Society of Thoracic Surgery (STS) database (7137 open, 4394 VATS) was significantly lower in the VATS group (6.7% VATS vs 9.3% open, $P<.001$). Licht and colleagues[21] used the Danish Lung Cancer Registry to confirm a similar result. In 1513 clinical stage I patients, both N1 upstaging (8.1% VATS vs 13.1% open, $P<.001$) and N2 upstaging (3.8% VATS vs 11.5% open, $P<.001$) were lower when patients were approached by VATS. The upstaging seen in the open groups of both these studies was more consistent with that seen in the large robotic series (**Table 3**). In neither study comparing VATS and thoracotomy were there differences in overall survival.

The cost of robotic technology in times of increasing health care expenditures is a real issue. Even without taking into consideration the amortized costs of these systems, robotics adds additional cost compared with conventional VATS.[22] However, a recent analysis of the voluntary STS database reported that although the percentage of all lobectomies performed by VATS has been increasing, overall, only 20% were performed by VATS during the 3-year study period ending in 2006.[10] Furthermore, there are some data, such as an even more recent analysis of a nonvoluntary national insurance database reporting that less than 6% of lobectomies were performed by VATS, that suggest that the overall adoption rate of VATS lobectomy may be lower in nonacademic, community-based settings.[11] If robotic technology can lead to greater adoption of a minimally invasive approach in a safe and appropriate manner,

the added cost may be justified by all the attendant benefits over traditional open surgery. Moreover, as use of robotic technology for thoracic surgical procedures increases, it will be important for future studies to attempt to discern differences between robotic and VATS approaches with respect to important outcomes, such as postoperative pain and quality of life.

SUMMARY

Robotic lobectomy is a feasible, safe, and oncologically sound surgical treatment of early-stage lung cancer. The technique is reproducible across multiple centers and in the long-term yields results consistent with the best seen with conventional VATS and thoracotomy. With respect to lymphadenectomy, there is evidence to suggest that it may reduce inadequate staging of the hilar and mediastinal nodes during curative, anatomic resection. Differences between robotic versus VATS versus thoracotomy approaches to thoracic diseases should be evaluated to define the appropriate role of each approach.

REFERENCES

1. Siegel S, Naishadam D, Jemal A. Cancer statistics, 2012. CA Cancer J Clin 2012;62:10–29.
2. National Lung Screening Trial Research Team, Aberle DR, Berg CD, et al. The National Lung Screening Trial: overview and study design. Radiology 2011;258:243–53.
3. McKenna RJ Jr, Houck W, Fuller CB. Video-assisted thoracic surgery lobectomy: experience with 1,100 cases. Ann Thorac Surg 2006;81:421–6.
4. Onaitis MW, Petersen RP, Balderson SS, et al. Thoracoscopic lobectomy is a safe and versatile procedure. Ann Surg 2006;244:420–5.

5. Flores RM, Park BJ, Dycoco J, et al. Lobectomy by video-assisted thoracic surgery (VATS) versus thoracotomy for lung cancer. J Thorac Cardiovasc Surg 2009;138:11–8.

6. Villamizar NR, Darrabie MD, Burfeind WR, et al. Thoracoscopic lobectomy is associated with lower morbidity compared with thoracotomy. J Thorac Cardiovasc Surg 2009;138:419–25.

7. Cattaneo SM, Park BJ, Wilton AS, et al. Use of video-assisted thoracic surgery for lobectomy in the elderly results in fewer complications. Ann Thorac Surg 2008;85:231–6.

8. Landreneau RJ, Hazelrigg SR, Mack MJ, et al. Postoperative pain-related morbidity: video-assisted thoracic surgery versus thoracotomy. Ann Thorac Surg 1993;56:1285–9.

9. Petersen RP, Pham D, Burfeind WR, et al. Thoracoscopic lobectomy facilitates the delivery of chemotherapy after resection for lung cancer. Ann Thorac Surg 2007;83:1245–50.

10. Boffa DJ, Allen MS, Grab JD, et al. Data from the Society of Thoracic Surgeons General Thoracic Surgery database: the surgical management of primary lung tumors. J Thorac Cardiovasc Surg 2008;135:247–54.

11. Gopaldas RR, Bakeen FG, Dao TK, et al. Video-assisted thoracoscopic versus open thoracotomy lobectomy in a cohort of 13,619 patients. Ann Thorac Surg 2010;89:1563–70.

12. Melfi FM, Ambrogi MC, Lucchi M, et al. Video robotic lobectomy. Multimed Man Cardiothorac Surg 2005. http://dx.doi.org/10.1510/mmcts.2004.000448.

13. Park BJ, Flores RM, Rusch VW. Robotic assistance for video-assisted thoracic surgical lobectomy: technique and initial results. J Thorac Cardiovasc Surg 2006;131:54–9.

14. Veronesi G, Galetta D, Maisonneuve P, et al. Four-arm robotic lobectomy for the treatment of early-stage lung cancer. J Thorac Cardiovasc Surg 2010;140:19–25.

15. Gharagozloo F, Margolis M, Tempesta B, et al. Robot-assisted lobectomy for early-stage lung cancer: report of 100 consecutive cases. Ann Thorac Surg 2009;88:380–4.

16. Cerfolio RJ, Bryant AS, Skylizard L, et al. Initial consecutive experience of completely portal robotic pulmonary resection with 4 arms. J Thorac Cardiovasc Surg 2011;142:740–6.

17. Park BJ, Melfi F, Mussi A, et al. Robotic lobectomy for non-small cell lung cancer (NSCLC): long-term oncologic results. J Thorac Cardiovasc Surg 2012;143:383–9.

18. Swanson SJ, Herndon JE, D'Amico TA, et al. Video-assisted thoracic surgery lobectomy: report of CALGB 39802-a prospective, multi-institutional feasibility trial. J Clin Oncol 2007;25:4993–7.

19. Goldstraw P, Crowley J, Chansky K, et al. The IASLC Lung Cancer Staging Project: proposals for the revision of the TNM stage groupings in the forthcoming (seventh) edition of the TNM classification of malignant tumours. J Thorac Oncol 2007;2:706–14.

20. Boffa DJ, Kosinski AS, Paul S, et al. Lymph node evaluation by open or video-assisted approaches in 11,500 anatomic lung cancer resections. Ann Thorac Surg 2012;94:347–53.

21. Licht PB, Jorgensen OD, Ladegaard L, et al. A national study of nodal upstaging after thoracoscopic versus open lobectomy for clinical stage I lung cancer. Ann Thorac Surg 2013;96:943–9.

22. Park BJ, Flores RM. Cost comparison of robotic, video-assisted thoracic surgery and thoracotomy approaches to pulmonary lobectomy. Thorac Surg Clin 2008;18:297–300.

Robot-assisted Lung Anatomic Segmentectomy: Technical Aspects

Alessandro Pardolesi, MD*, Giulia Veronesi, MD

KEYWORDS

- Anatomic lung segmentectomy • Robot-assisted lung resection
- Early stage non–small cell lung cancer

KEY POINTS

- Robot-assisted anatomic lung segmentectomy for non–small cell lung cancer and lung metastases is feasible and safe.
- Segmentectomy allows assessment of hilar, bronchial, and vascular lymph nodes, which is important because lymph nodes can be involved even in clinical stage IA disease.
- With increasing use of lung cancer screening for high-risk individuals, more small early stage lung cancers will be detected.
- Robotic surgical systems have several advantages compared with traditional video-assisted thoracoscopic surgery, including three-dimensional field of view and more degrees of movement freedom for robotic arms, which replicate human arm and wrist movements.

 Videos of upper segmentectomy right lower lobe, upper segmentectomy left lower lobe and trisegmentectomy of left upper lobe (lingula-sparing lobectomy) accompany this article at http://www.thoracic.theclinics.com/

INTRODUCTION

With the widespread use of computed tomography (CT) and the potential adoption of low-dose CT lung cancer screening for high-risk individuals, it is expected that the number of small early stage lung cancers diagnosed will increase. The optimal treatment of these small lesions may not be lobectomy, and extended or anatomic segmentectomy[1–3] as well wedge resection[4] have been investigated for small (<2 cm), stage I lung cancers, particularly those that present as ground-glass opacities.[3,4] However the Lung Cancer Study Group randomized trial,[5] which compared lobectomy with limited resection (segmentectomy and wedge), found significantly more local recurrences and deaths in patients receiving limited resection than lobectomy. The increased adverse events were mainly evident in patients receiving wedge resection.

Although wedge resection is removal of a small wedge-shaped portion of the lung, anatomic segmentectomy is excision of one or more of the bronchopulmonary segments of a lung lobe, with ligation and division of each of the bronchi and of the blood vessels serving the segments. In addition, and unlike wedge resection, segmentectomy involves assessment of hilar, bronchial, and vascular lymph nodes, which is important because, even with clinical stage IA disease, lymph nodes can be involved. Proponents of limited surgery for primary lung cancer insist that adequate lymph node assessment for staging is

The authors have nothing to disclose.
Division of Thoracic Surgery, European Institute of Oncology, Via Ripamonti 435, Milano 20141, Italy
* Corresponding author.
E-mail address: alessandro.pardolesi@ieo.it

Thorac Surg Clin 24 (2014) 163–168
http://dx.doi.org/10.1016/j.thorsurg.2014.02.008
1547-4127/14/$ – see front matter © 2014 Elsevier Inc. All rights reserved.

a crucial aspect of the surgical procedure.[6] Some single-arm studies have reported that 5-year and disease-free survival for segmentectomy are indistinguishable from survival for lobectomy in patients with early stage lung cancer with lesions less than 2 cm.[7–9]

In patients with secondary lung cancer eligible for surgery, anatomic segmentectomy may be beneficial as a way of optimizing future resection. In such cases, hilar node dissection often uncovers occult nodal involvement when the metastases are centrally located.

Anatomic segmentectomy can be performed by open surgery or minimally invasive video-assisted thoracic surgery (VATS). However VATS is technically demanding because the surgeon has restricted ability to maneuver the instruments, only two-dimensional visualization, and has lost the eye-hand-target axis. VATS is therefore performed by a small number of highly experienced groups, and few publications on segmentectomy performed by VATS are available.[10,11,12]

The theoretic advantages of robotic thoracic surgery compared with VATS include high-definition stereoscopic visualization; greater dexterity, because the robotic arms replicate human arm and wrist movements and provide more degrees of movement freedom; no fulcrum effect; filtration of physiologic tremor; and greater comfort for the surgeon (**Box 1**).[13]

This article describes the robotic technique we use in Milan to perform robot-assisted anatomic lung segmentectomy for early stage lung cancer and lung metastases, and present early outcomes.

SURGICAL TECHNIQUE
Preoperative Planning

Preoperative work-up includes chest CT, standard hematology and blood chemistry, cardiologic examination, and assessment of pulmonary function. Positron emission tomography (PET) CT may be useful in selected cases. Patients with evidence of a single lesion considered resectable

by segmentectomy are eligible for robot-assisted surgery.

Robot Preparation and Patient Positioning

Operating room staff set up the robot console and visual system. All procedures are performed under general anesthesia. Patients are placed in lateral decubitus with the hips flexed and secured by fixing the pelvis as shown in **Fig. 1**. One-lung ventilation is achieved by the use of a double-lumen endotracheal tube. The robot is positioned at the head of the patient (**Fig. 2**).

Port Placement

The operation begins by making a 1-cm incision for the camera (30° stereoscopic instrument). The camera is inserted to explore the thoracic cavity and, at this point in the procedure, to provide visual guidance for the 3-cm utility incision, which is made at the fourth or fifth intercostal space anteriorly. Next, an 8-mm incision is made at the eighth intercostal space in the posterior axillary line. The fourth incision made posteriorly in the auscultatory triangle and allows lung retraction and hence better field exposure. Port placement varies little with the type of segmentectomy and side; however, for left-side operations, the camera port is placed more laterally than for the right side so that the heart does not obscure the operating field (**Figs. 3–5**).

Posterior Segmentectomy, Right Upper Lobe

The lung is retracted anteriorly. The first step is dissection of the interlobar portion of the pulmonary artery so as to identify the junction between the posterior ascending and lower lobe superior segmental arteries. It is helpful to excise the interlobar lymph nodes. The posterior portion of the major fissure is divided either by cautery or by stapler. The ascending branch is then isolated and ligated either with an endovascular stapler or a cut between robotic clips. The upper lobe is pulled

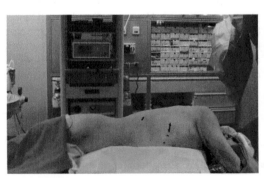

Fig. 1. Patient positioning.

Box 1
Benefits of robotic surgery compared with minimally invasive thoracic surgery

- Three-dimensional view
- Improved ergonomics
- Stable camera platform
- Elimination of tremor
- EndoWrist technology

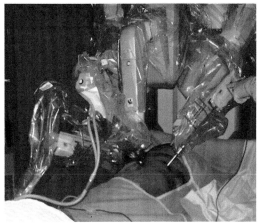

Fig. 2. Robot positioning. The robot is positioned at the head of the patient. (*Courtesy of* Intuitive Surgical Intuitive Surgical, Sunnyvale, CA; with permission.)

anteriorly, to expose the division of the upper lobe and intermediate bronchi. The peribronchial tissue is dissected distally to expose the posterior segmental bronchus, which is encircled and divided by the stapler. Next, the posterior segmental vein is identified, isolated, and divided. The segmental fissures are divided with multiple firings of the endoscopic stapler.

Anterior Segmentectomy, Right Upper Lobe

The mediastinal pleura is incised anteriorly from the middle lobe vein to the truncus arteriosus.

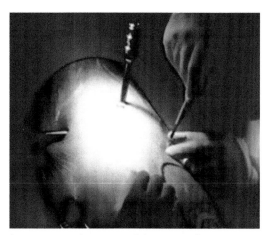

Fig. 4. Trocar placement, right approach.

The anterior segmental vein is isolated and divided. Next, the anterior segmental artery coming from the lower portion of the truncus is isolated and divided. The anterior portion of the horizontal fissure is completed with an endovascular stapler, and the anterior segmental bronchus is isolated and divided. The remaining segmental fissures are divided with the stapler.

Upper Segmentectomy, Right or Left Lower Lobe

The inferior pulmonary ligament is divided up to the pulmonary vein. Distal dissection of the vein

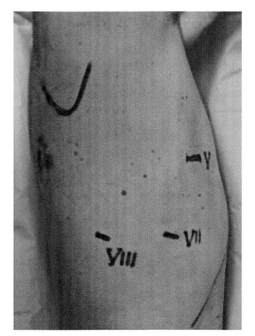

Fig. 3. Port placement, right approach.

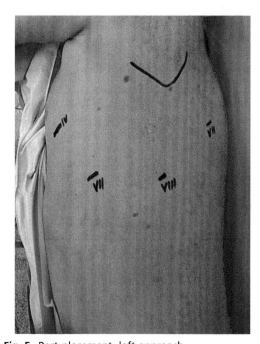

Fig. 5. Port placement, left approach.

posteriorly exposes the superior segmental vein, which is ligated with the endovascular stapler (Videos 1 and 2). After division of the vein, the bronchus is isolated with the lung still retracted anteriorly. The lower lobe apical segmental artery in the fissure is then identified and stapled or clipped. The last step is transection of the parenchyma, with the stapler introduced through the utility incision. The operating technique for upper segmentectomy of the left lower lobe is similar.

Trisegmentectomy of Left Upper Lobe (Lingula-sparing Lobectomy)

The mediastinal pleura is incised over the superior vein, and the branches superior to the lingular branch are isolated and divided using the stapler (Video 3). The anterior branch of the pulmonary artery is isolated and divided, allowing mobilization of the upper lobe bronchus and sparing of the lingular branch of the pulmonary artery. Once the anterior branch of the pulmonary artery is stapled, the remaining apicoposterior branches are isolated and ligated with an anterior or posterior approach. The fissure is stapled last.

Lingulectomy

The mediastinal pleura is divided over the lingular vein, which is divided between clips or by the endovascular stapler. The interlobar pleura is divided over the basilar pulmonary artery to expose the lingular branch. The anterior fissure is divided by cautery or stapler. The lingular pulmonary artery is isolated and divided, exposing the lingular bronchus. Once the bronchus is divided, the fissures are completed by the stapler.

Basilar Segmentectomy of Left or Right Lower Lobe

The inferior pulmonary ligament is divided to the level of the inferior pulmonary vein. Distal dissection is performed to expose the basilar vein, sparing the branch to the superior segment. The vein is divided and dissection continued in the anterior portion of the major fissure. The mediastinal pleura is divided to expose the basilar pulmonary artery; the anterior part of the fissure is divided to expose the bronchus. The basal pulmonary artery is stapled, and the basal bronchus is isolated and also stapled. The fissures are completed last.

Mediastinal Lymph Node Dissection

Lymph node dissection is performed with the trocars and camera port in their usual positions. The hook is usually manipulated by the surgeon's right hand and the forceps by the left hand,

irrespective of the side of approach. The other Cadière forceps (Intuitive Surgical, Sunnyvale, CA), the fourth robotic arm, is used for lung retraction and positioning. An Ultracision PK system (PK Technology G400 Generator, Gyrus ACMI LP, Maple Grove, MN) or bipolar forceps is occasionally used instead of the monopolar hook. A metal suction tube is introduced by the assistant through the anterior incision below the robotic arm, and is used to evacuate smoke and blood, and to provide occasional retraction. Complete dissection or sampling of the nodes is usually performed at the end of the lung procedure. For primary lung cancer, if regional and mediastinal nodes are enlarged (>1 cm) they are sent for intraoperative frozen section to rule out metastatic nodal disease. For culmen or lingular resections, lymph node dissection of the pulmonary window is performed first to facilitate dissection of the branches of the pulmonary artery and of the upper pulmonary vein. Hilar lymphadenectomy is performed while the hilum is being dissected.

IMMEDIATE POSTOPERATIVE CARE

On completion of surgery, patients are extubated and pass 1 or 2 hours in the recovery room with cardiorespiratory monitoring. They are then transferred to the ward. Cardiorespiratory function, blood pressure, temperature, urine output, and hemoglobin saturation are monitored while in the ward. A chest radiograph is performed shortly after the end of the procedure.

REHABILITATION AND RECOVERY

If there are no complications requiring specific treatment or intensive care, patients are mobilized and start eating on the first postoperative day. Intravenous fluid administration is generally maintained during the first 24 hours. Prophylactic antibiotics, started before surgery, are administered for not more than 72 hours, even if the chest tube remains in place.

Postoperative pain is usually well controlled by a combination of local anesthetic (bupivacaine or ropivacaine infiltrated into the wounds), subcutaneous morphine (5 or 10 mg every 4 or 6 hours), and intravenous paracetamol (every 6 hours). The chest tube(s) is removed on the second or third postoperative day providing not more than 250 mL of fluid are collected over 24 hours, there is no air leak, and the lung is appears to be completely expanded on the chest radiograph. Patients undergo intensive lung rehabilitation starting on the first postoperative day and continuing until discharge.

Table 1
Characteristics of 17 patients who underwent robotic lung segmentectomy at the Memorial Sloan-Kettering Cancer Center, European Institute of Oncology, and Hackensack University Medical Center between January 2008 and December 2010

Variable	Number	Percentage
Age (y); mean (range)	68.2 (32–82)	—
Sex (M/F)	7/10	41.2/58.8
Tumor size (cm); mean (range)	1.11 (0.6–2.8)	—
Segmentectomy location/type		
Left lower lobe superior	4	23.5
Right lower lobe superior	3	17.6
Lingulectomy	3	17.6
Left upper lobe trisegmentectomy (lingula sparing)	2	11.9
Left lower lobe basal	4	23.5
Right upper lobe anterior	1	5.9
Primary lung cancer histology	10	58.8
Adenocarcinoma	5	—
Squamous cell carcinoma	1	—
Bronchioloalveolar carcinoma	2	—
Typical carcinoid	2	—
Secondary lung cancer	7	41.2

CLINICAL RESULTS IN THE LITERATURE

Seventeen consecutive patients underwent robotic lung segmentectomy at the Memorial Sloan-Kettering Cancer Center (New York), European Institute of Oncology (Milan, Italy), and Hackensack University Medical Center (New Jersey) from January 1, 2008, to December 1 2010. Ten were women, 7 were men. Mean age was 68.2 years (range 32–82 years). Mean operating time was 189 minutes (range 138–240 minutes) (**Table 1**).[14]

Most lesions (64.7%) affected the lower lobe. There were no conversions to either VATS or thoracotomy. Median postoperative stay was 5 days (range 2–14 days). Postoperative mortality was 0%. Early postoperative complications (17.6%) were minor: 1 (5.9%) pneumonia, 2 prolonged air leaks (11.9%). In 5 patients (29.4%) the diagnosis was obtained before surgery by fine-needle aspiration biopsy. Final pathology identified non–small cell lung cancer in 8 patients, typical carcinoid in 2, and lung metastases in 7. The metastases were histologically compatible with colon carcinoma in 3 patients, and breast cancer, gastrointestinal trophoblastic tumor adenoid cystic carcinoma, and osteogenic sarcoma in 1 patient each.

Two of the primary lung cancers were pN1 and 6 were pN0. Median tumor size was 1.11 cm (range 0.6–2.8 cm). PET was performed in 12 cases; it was nor performed in 5 cases with clinically suspected of lung metastases. PET was considered positive (visual assessment) in 9 (75%) cases.

SUMMARY

Initial experience of anatomic robotic segmentectomy in patients with a single primary or metastatic lung lesion is encouraging. No major complications and no conversion to open surgery were reported, operating times were acceptable, and hospital stay was in line with that for VATS lung procedures.[8] Anatomic robotic segmentectomy seems to offer all the advantages of minimally invasive surgery and provides the additional advantages of greater dexterity, three-dimensional vision, and greater surgeon comfort, thereby facilitating precise anatomic dissection, including lymphadenectomy, which promises to be oncologically radical. However, further studies are required to compare robotic segmentectomy with open and VATS approaches, and long-term follow-up is necessary to verify the oncologic efficacy of the robotic technique. If the advantages are confirmed by experience, it is expected that robotic procedures will be more widely adopted by thoracic surgeons than the more demanding VATS, even though the high cost of robotic units remains a problem. However, robotic technology is evolving quickly, and costs may decrease as the technology matures, competing manufacturers enter the field,

Box 2
Summary

- Screening results in increased diagnosis of very early stage lung cancer disease
- Survival benefit of minimally invasive versus open procedures
- Randomized controlled trial ongoing in United States and Japan comparing limited resection with lobectomy for lung cancer for stage 1a disease less than 2 cm
- Robotic segmentectomy is feasible and safe
- Robotic technology has simplified complex minimally invasive procedures
- Future task: to show the superiority of robotics versus VATS

and more machines become available. The introduction of robotic staplers, aspirators, and 5-mm lung forceps will further increase precision (**Box 2**).

SUPPLEMENTARY DATA

Videos related to this article can be found online at http://dx.doi.org/10.1016/j.thorsurg.2014.02.008.

REFERENCES

1. Yoshikawa K, Tsubota N, Kodama K, et al. Prospective study of extended segmentectomy for small lung tumors: the final report. Ann Thorac Surg 2002;73:1055–9.
2. Kodama K, Doi O, Higashiyama M, et al. Intentional limited resection for selected patients with T1 N0 M0 non-small-cell lung cancer: a single-institution study. J Thorac Cardiovasc Surg 1997;114:347–53.
3. Jensik RJ, Faber LP, Kittle CF. Segmental resection for bronchogenic carcinoma. Ann Thorac Surg 1979;28:475–83.
4. Peters RM. The role of limited resection in carcinoma of the lung. Am J Surg 1982;143:706–10.
5. Ginberg RJ, Rubinstein LV. Randomized trial of lobectomy versus limited resection for T1 N0 non-small cell lung cancer. Ann Thorac Surg 1995;60: 615–23.
6. Keenan RJ, Landreneau RJ, Maley RH, et al. Segmental resection spares pulmonary function in patients with stage 1 lung cancer. Ann Thorac Surg 2004;78:228–33.
7. Harada H, Okada M, Sakamoto T, et al. Functional advantage after radical segmentectomy versus lobectomy for lung cancer. Ann Thorac Surg 2005; 80:2041–5.
8. Okada M, Yoshikawa K, Hatta T, et al. Is segmentectomy with lymph node assessment an alternative to lobectomy for non-small cell lung cancer of 2 cm or smaller? Ann Thorac Surg 2001;71: 956–61.
9. Koike T, Yamato Y, Yoshiya K, et al. Intentional limited pulmonary resection for peripheral T1 N0 M0 small-sized lung cancer. J Thorac Cardiovasc Surg 2003;125:924–8.
10. Petersen RP, Pham D, Burfeind WR, et al. Thoracoscopic lobectomy facilitates the delivery of chemotherapy after resection for lung cancer. Ann Thorac Surg 2007;83:1245–9.
11. Atkins BZ, Harpole DH, Magnum JH, et al. Pulmonary segmentectomy by thoracotomy or thoracoscopy: reduced hospital length of stay with a minimally-invasive approach. Ann Thorac Surg 2007;84:1107–12.
12. Whitson BA, Groth SS, Duval SJ, et al. Surgery for early-stage non-small cell lung cancer: a systematic review of the video-assisted thoracoscopic surgery versus thoracotomy approaches to lobectomy. Ann Thorac Surg 2008;86(6):2008–16. http://dx.doi.org/10.1016/j.athoracsur.2008.07.009 [discussion: 2016–8].
13. Veronesi G. Robotic surgery for the treatment of early-stage lung cancer. Curr Opin Oncol 2013; 25(2):107–14.
14. Pardolesi A, Park B, Petrella F, et al. Robotic anatomic segmentectomy of the lung: technical aspects and initial results. Ann Thorac Surg 2012;94(3):929–34. http://dx.doi.org/10.1016/j.athoracsur.2012.04.086.

Robotic Pneumonectomy

Brian E. Louie, MD, MHA, MPH, FRCSC, FACS

KEYWORDS

- Robotic • Pneumonectomy • Video-assisted thoracoscopy • Lung cancer

KEY POINTS

- Pneumonectomy is considered when a lung-preserving operation is deemed inadequate.
- There is little published experience with robotic pneumonectomy.
- Hilar nodal dissection facilitates access to the three main vascular structures with order of division: superior vein, main artery, and inferior vein.
- Robotic pneumonectomy is an advanced robotic procedure that requires considerable prior robotic experience.

INTRODUCTION: NATURE OF THE PROBLEM

Over the last two decades, minimally invasive lobectomy by video-assisted thoracic surgery (VATS) and more recently robotic assistance has become routine in many centers around the world for early stage non–small cell lung cancer. These minimally invasive techniques have been shown to result in improved postoperative outcomes, such as blood loss and length of stay[1]; to provide equivalent oncologic outcomes[2]; and to be superior for elderly patients[3] and those with reduced pulmonary function.[4] Despite this evidence, recent estimates show that 70% of lobectomies for clinical stage I cancers are still performed by thoracotomy in the highly selected Society for Thoracic Surgeon's database[5] and 6% in the Nationwide Inpatient Sample database.[6] Thus, the idea of approaching a patient who may require a pneumonectomy using VATS or robotic-assisted techniques is likely to be met with some skepticism, a lot of vehemence and hesitation, and disapproving looks from many thoracic surgeons.

Although there has been a rapid expansion in the use of robotic-assisted lung resection, the published experience remains small and limited to several pioneering centers. To date the most advanced centers have produced reports on lobectomy[7–11] and segmentectomy.[12] Outside of two case reports[13,14] there have been no published series on robotic pneumonectomy. This article discusses the indications for minimally invasive pneumonectomy; reviews the robotic set up, surgical approaches, and techniques; discusses the potential benefits and disadvantages of the robotic approach; and suggests a future role of robotic pneumonectomy.

SURGICAL TECHNIQUE
Indications and Patient Selection

The indications for pneumonectomy are the same regardless of approach. The two most common include usually a centrally placed non–small cell lung cancer or extensive hilar nodal disease encasing the proximal hilar structures, particularly the pulmonary artery. Other indications such as synchronous, multilobar disease or metachronous disease in the remaining lobe are less common. Our approach to centrally located lesions is to first attempt to perform a lung-preserving operation, such as a bronchial and/or vascular sleeve resection and consider pneumonectomy as a backup option should lung preservation be ruled out as an option during initial exploration. Because of the relatively uncommon absolute indications to perform pneumonectomy and the potential morbidity regardless of approach, patients should be carefully selected

Disclosure: The author discloses he is was on the speaker's bureau and a surgical proctor for Intuitive Surgical.
Minimally Invasive Thoracic Surgery Program, Division of Thoracic Surgery, Swedish Cancer Institute and Medical Center, Suite 900, 1101 Madison Street, Seattle, WA 98104, USA
E-mail address: brian.louie@swedish.org

Thorac Surg Clin 24 (2014) 169–175
http://dx.doi.org/10.1016/j.thorsurg.2014.02.007
1547-4127/14/$ – see front matter © 2014 Elsevier Inc. All rights reserved.

both from the standpoint of oncologic need and operative risk. As a result, experience with robotic pneumonectomy is and will remain limited. However, there are instances when this procedure may be indicated and performance via a minimally invasive approach may confer significant benefits perioperatively to patients.

Preoperative Planning

Preoperative planning for all of our lung resections is similar and includes diagnostic computed tomography of the chest to include the adrenal glands, combined computed tomography/positron emission tomography imaging, and pulmonary function tests. For centrally placed tumors where there is a possibility of pneumonectomy, these patients undergo magnetic resonance imaging of the brain, quantitative ventilation-perfusion scan when required, and cardiac evaluation with at least echocardiogram. Bronchoscopy with biopsy and mediastinoscopy is typically performed several days before resection. It is our strong preference to have a confirmed tissue diagnosis before exploration in patients where pneumonectomy is a possibility to minimize any need for intraoperative biopsy.

Preparation and Patient Positioning

Patients are positioned similarly to all open or VATS procedures with the patient in lateral decubitus position following endotracheal intubation and establishment of single lung ventilation. For robotic cases, the operating room table is reversed to put the patient's head at the foot of the bed to allow for positioning of the robot and to allow for the patient's hip to be level with the chest or below (**Fig. 1**). This positioning allows the robotic camera to move freely from anterior to posterior without catching on the hip. Anesthesia is positioned to the face side of the patient to facilitate access to

the double-lumen tube and the robot is positioned over the patient's head. If the bed is not reversed, the robot is positioned with the center column just behind the patient's head at an angle of 10 to 45 degrees from the axis of the patient.[13]

Multiple arm set ups for robotic lung resection have been described. The three-arm with utility incision[13] and a completely portal four-arm approach[14] have been used to complete robotic pneumonectomy.

Three-arm set up

The three-arm set up we currently use has the camera arm and robotic arms 1 and 3 with the number 2 arm stored (**Fig. 2**). The initial 8-mm port is placed in the sixth interspace posterior axillary line and is used with robotic arm 1. Using the robotic 8-mm camera, the remaining ports are placed under direct visualization based on internal anatomy and external position in the following order: 12-mm camera port along the line between the scapular tip and the anterior superior iliac spine to enter the chest at the top of the diaphragm seen internally, which usually coincides with the eighth or ninth interspace and an 8-mm robotic arm 3 inferior and posterior to the scapular tip at the level of the superior segment. A 12-mm laparoscopic port placed in the midaxillary line to enter the chest

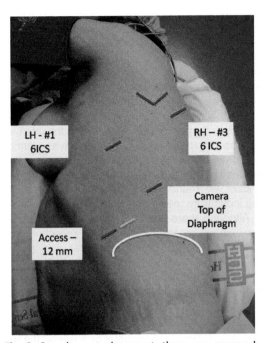

Fig. 2. Sample port placement: three-arm approach. *Yellow curve* indicates the diaphragm, *Red lines* indicates the port sites, *Red "v"* indicates the scapular tip, *Green line* indicates the extension of extraction incision.

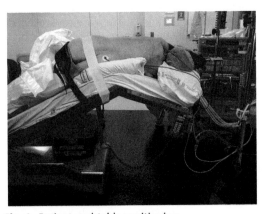

Fig. 1. Patient and table positioning.

just at the diaphragmatic insertion is the fourth port and used for retraction, stapling, and suctioning by the bedside assistant. Alternatively, a 4-cm utility incision can be placed in the fourth interspace anteriorly instead of the fourth port to facilitate suctioning and stapling by a bedside assistant.

Carbon dioxide insufflation is administered to a pressure of 6 to 8 mm Hg with a flow of 6 to 8 mL/min until the lung is deflated and then stopped. Four robotic instruments are used: (1) Cadiere forceps, (2) fenestrated bipolar, (3) curved bipolar dissector, and (4) L hook. Through the 12-mm port either a laparoscopic forceps is used retraction without grasping the lung or a suction-irrigation device is introduced. The specimen is placed in an extraction bag and removed by enlarging the camera port to approximately 5 cm.

Four-arm set up (Completely Portal Robotic Lobectomy-4)

In a completely portal robotic lobectomy-4 (CPRL-4) robotic lobectomy, a total of five ports are placed but all three robotic arms are used (**Fig. 3**). The port placement for these is based on work by Cerfolio and colleagues.[7] In this approach, the pleural space is entered with a 5-mm port anteriorly in the midaxillary line at the top rib seven. CO_2 insufflation is also used in

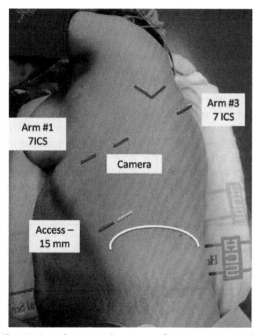

Fig. 3. Sample port placement: four-arm approach. *Yellow curve* indicates the diaphragm, *Red lines* indicates the port sites, *Red "v"* indicates the scapular tip, *Green line* indicates the extension of extraction incision.

this approach. A 5-mm VATS camera is inserted to placement of the remaining ports based on internal anatomy. The most posterior port (5 mm, arm 3) is placed two rib spaces below the major fissure and just above the angle of the rib. Once this interspace is selected, all other ports are positioned in the same interspace moving from posterior to anterior as follows: arm 2 is an 8-mm port placed 10 cm from the initial port; camera port is an 8- or 12-mm port placed 9 cm from arm 2; arm 1 is a 12-mm port placed 9 cm anterior to the camera port. A 15-mm access port is placed in the ninth interspace mid to anterior axillary line. Stapling is performed by the 15-mm access port or by removing the instrument in arm 1. The specimen is extracted by enlarging the 15-mm port to approximately 5 cm.

Surgical Procedure

The exact steps of the operation are surgeon and tumor dependent. However, two reports of robotic pneumonectomy have provided some insights into the conduct of the operation.[13,14]

The initial steps in both reports were similar. After division of the inferior pulmonary ligament, exposure and isolation of the superior and inferior pulmonary veins is accomplished followed by exposure of the central pulmonary artery. In our experience this is facilitated at the inferior vein by removal of station 9 lymph nodes and at the superior vein by dissecting out the hilar lymph nodes. The hilar dissection and inferior vein exposure is also facilitated by exploration of the subcarinal space and removal of the station 7 lymph node packet. On the right, this dissection helps to isolate the right main stem bronchus.

After the vessels are isolated, the veins are divided first to allow exposure and access to the pulmonary artery, which was the last vessel divided. However, Spaggiari and Galetta[13] noted that engorgement of the lung occurred using this sequence of vessel division making the pneumonectomy more difficult. In their second pneumonectomy they divided the upper vein first followed by the artery. The inferior vein was divided last and the degree of engorgement was noted to be less.

Division of the main bronchus on the right was uncomplicated. However, two of the reported robotic pneumonectomies were left sided. Division of the left main stem bronchus to achieve a short stump was identified as providing an inherent challenge with the need to overcome the aortic arch. Both authors noted the need for significant retraction on the lung. One used an umbilical tape to achieve retraction, whereas the other withdrew the double lumen and advanced the bronchial lumen into the right main stem. Roticulating linear staplers (45 and 60 mm) were also required to achieve as short a stump as possible.

Retrieval of the lung was accomplished through a standard 4-cm incision in all three cases with the aid of a specimen retrieval sac. However, both authors did note that "gentle" rotary motions and "patient maneuvers" were required for extraction.

Although this is a general approach, the exact steps are dictated by the location and size of the tumor and the patient's anatomy.

Immediate Postoperative Care

The immediate postoperative care of a pneumonectomy is the same at our center regardless of the surgical approach. Patients are usually extubated in the operating room. The mediastinum is balanced by placing a single chest tube with the tip in the midthoracic cavity. The chest tube is connected to tubing that is draped up over an intravenous pole and above the patient's shoulder and connected to a water seal device without suction. Provided the mediastinum is balanced and there is no bleeding, the tube is removed the next day.

CLINICAL RESULTS IN THE LITERATURE

At the present time, a total of six robotic pneumonectomies (**Table 1**) have been attempted, only four were completed using robotic assistance, and three provided technical details of the procedure. There were two conversions: one for "oncologic reasons" and the other for a right-sided central pulmonary artery injury that led to death on postoperative day 17. It seems that each of the surgeons had accumulated a "reasonable" experience with robotic lung resection with the range of cases between 38 and 154; however, only Spaggiari and Galetta[13] indicated the prior case experience with lobectomy before they attempted the pneumonectomy. The limited length of stay and follow-up data are similar to open pneumonectomy.

Access to and division of the central pulmonary artery is arguably the most important step in conducting the operation particularly because the operating surgeon is at the console, and one of the attempted robotic pneumonectomy patients died from an injury to the pulmonary artery.[15] In our lobectomy experience, we found that completing the nodal dissection in the mediastinum and the hilum facilitated division of the vessels. Complete exposure of both pulmonary veins and the main pulmonary artery are necessary to robotic pneumonectomy. On the right, division of the superior vein is necessary to access the truncus and the main artery (**Fig. 4**). Division of the truncus arteriosis was a necessary step in VATS pneumonectomy because it allowed access to the main artery in a more accessible spot.[16] Similarly, on the left, resection of the aorto-pulmonary window tissue and division of the superior vein provide better access to the main left artery (**Fig. 5**).[16] A vessel loop or large-gauge ligature placed around the artery is helpful to narrow the arterial diameter and facilitate stapler placement.

Management of the main bronchus, particularly the left, seems to pose a challenge during robotic pneumonectomy. The need to have a short left-sided bronchial stump has been well described as have the complications attributed to a long stump. In both case reports, there was a need to place considerable traction on the left lung to overcome the aortic arch. Then, roticulating linear staplers up to 60 mm in size were used to divide the bronchus. In the open approach, we have found using a linear stapler sometimes works but often we default to a TA style stapler to gain better access. With such limited experience it is difficult to anticipate whether these linear staplers will always be able to achieve a short stump especially if the length of the left main is underestimated by the magnification of the minimally invasive approaches.[17] One suggestion to improve access to the left main was to withdraw the left-sided double-lumen tube and advance the bronchial tip into the right lung to allow more mobility to ensure a short stump.[14] Our experience with this technique has not been as helpful. Lastly,

Table 1
Approaches and outcomes of robotic pneumonectomy

Author	# Robotic Cases	N	Side	Approach	Length of Stay (d)	Morbidity	Follow-up (m)
Giulianotti et al,[15] 2010	38	3	—	Three-arm/utility	—	Two converted, one death (pulmonary artery bleed)	—
Dylewski et al,[8] 2011	154	1	—	Three-arm/utility	—	—	—
Spaggiari et al, 2011	54	2	R/L	Three-arm/utility	6.5	None	15
Rodriguez,[14] 2013	—	1	L	Four-arm	4	None	—

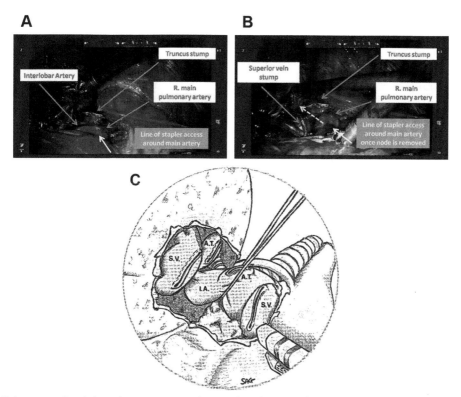

Fig. 4. (*A*) Access to the right pulmonary artery shown after division of the truncus arteriosis. (*B*) Access to the right pulmonary artery showing line of access once the lymph node at the inferior edge of the artery is removed. (*C*) Diagram of right pulmonary artery anatomy. AT, truncus anterior; IA, intermediate artery; SV, superior pulmonary vein. (*From* Roviaro G, Varoli F, Vergani C, et al. Techniques of pneumonectomy. Video-assisted thoracic surgery pneumonectomy. Chest Surg Clin N Am 1999;9(2):430, xi–xii; with permission.)

achieving a short stump may become even harder particularly as patients who have undergone induction therapy, which can render the mediastinum less mobile, are approached robotically and require a pneumonectomy.

Extraction of the specimen through a 5-cm access incision seems like it should be a challenge. However, by leading with the apex of the upper lobe or an edge of the lower lobe rather than the hilum of the lung it is thought to be easily extracted with a rocking motion. Similar issues occurred during VATS pneumonectomy prompting several suggestions, such as suctioning the lung to induce atelectasis before stapling, piecemeal extraction, or lobar separation.[17] The ease of extraction may also be related to lung engorgement. Not only does engorgement obscure the view during robotic resection but it makes extraction difficult. Spaggiari and Galetta[13] suggest leaving the inferior vein intact until the main artery is divided to avoid this problem.

One issue that has not been addressed in any of the reports is how easy or difficult it is to adequately assess whether a lung-preserving operation could be performed. Bronchoscopic and histologic evaluation of the distal bronchi, as in the case reported by Rodriguez,[14] may predetermine the need for pneumonectomy. However, intraoperative assessment for tumors crossing fissures or vascular invasion may be the most difficult to assess and may best be assessed by thoracotomy. This might allow combining a lobectomy with segmentectomy or a bilobectomy to avoid the pneumonectomy and result in similar survival or to determine if sleeve vascular resection can be performed.

Given the present data available, the benefits of robotic or even VATS pneumonectomy are unclear. Early papers on VATS pneumonectomy suggested favorable short-term results and called for longer-term outcome data.[18] Only one center has provided longer-term data and compared it with open pneumonectomy.[19] The VATS group faired favorably in blood loss, intensive care unit stay, and overall length of stay when compared with open cases. However, 8 (25%) of 32 cases were converted from VATS to open. These conversions were for more advanced disease (five), fibrosis (two), and bleeding (one). This converted group

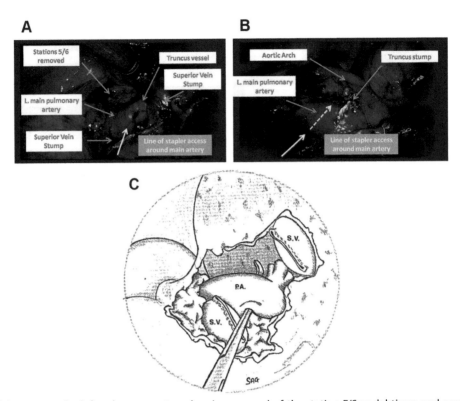

Fig. 5. (*A*) Access to the left pulmonary artery showing removal of the station 5/6 nodal tissue and proximity to the truncus branch and after vein division. (*B*) Access to the left pulmonary artery with the aortic arch identified and the truncus divided to facilitate access. (*C*) Diagram of left pulmonary artery anatomy. PA, pulmonary artery; SV, superior pulmonary vein. (*From* Roviaro G, Varoli F, Vergani C, et al. Techniques of pneumonectomy. Video-assisted thoracic surgery pneumonectomy. Chest Surg Clin N Am 1999;9(2):428, xi–xii; with permission.)

also had statistically worse outcomes than if they were to start with open pneumonectomy with greater blood loss, longer intensive care unit stay, and overall length of stay.

It is possible that robotic pneumonectomy may have similar results to this single institution VATS series. However, these series[13,14,19] do highlight two important issues.

First, how is a lung-preserving operation ruled out. In the VATS pneumonectomy series, 5 (22%) of 24 had stage I disease and 14 (61%) of 24 had stage II disease, and even though the authors state that the cases were not amenable to sleeve resection, there is no description in this series or the robotic case reports of how they determined a lung-preserving operation was not possible at thoracoscopy. In an open operation, a series of steps would be taken to determine the necessity of pneumonectomy, such as dissecting out the fissures and hilum to expose the pertinent vascular anatomy. In many cases the decision is made after several hours of dissecting and dividing several key structures or even cutting the bronchus and obtaining frozen sections. We firmly believe that the patient's outcome may be improved if a lung-

preserving operation is performed[20] compared with pneumonectomy and find it difficult to ascertain if lung preservation is feasible robotically given our current experience. Future reports should outline how the decision to proceed with pneumonectomy is determined.

Second, the reported conversion rate of 25% is expected and surgeons attempting robotic pneumonectomy should expect a similar experience during the learning curve. However, the operative outcomes for those being converted after a VATS attempt were significantly worse than if the operation had begun open. There are likely multiple factors resulting in these outcomes, but as the indications for robotic lung resection are broadened and experience is gained, clinicians must guard against worse outcomes in those patients requiring conversion.

SUMMARY

Although considerable experience has been gained with robotic lung resection, particularly lobectomy and segmentectomy, robotic pneumonectomy is an operation that is still undergoing development. In centers that have pioneered robotic lung surgery, lobectomy has reached a point where several standard approaches are done and the operation is undergoing optimization. Robotic pneumonectomy requires further development particularly around the ability to assess the need for lung-preserving surgery, optimal techniques for management of the pulmonary artery, and technology to address the bronchial length on the left. Until further experiences are gained, robotic pneumonectomy should be reserved for centers with considerable experience.

REFERENCES

1. Paul S, Altorki NK, Sheng S, et al. Thoracoscopic lobectomy is associated with lower morbidity than open lobectomy: a propensity-matched analysis from the STS database. J Thorac Cardiovasc Surg 2010;139(2):366–78.
2. Yan TD, Black D, Bannon PG, et al. Systematic review and meta-analysis of randomized and nonrandomized trials on safety and efficacy of video-assisted thoracic surgery lobectomy for early-stage non-small-cell lung cancer. J Clin Oncol 2009;27(15):2553–62.
3. Port JL, Mirza FM, Lee PC, et al. Lobectomy in octogenarians with non-small cell lung cancer: ramifications of increasing life expectancy and the benefits of minimally invasive surgery. Ann Thorac Surg 2011;92(6):1951–7.
4. Nakata M, Saeki H, Yokoyama N, et al. Pulmonary function after lobectomy: video-assisted thoracic surgery versus thoracotomy. Ann Thorac Surg 2000;70(3):938–41.
5. Boffa DJ, Kosinski AS, Paul S, et al. Lymph node evaluation by open or video-assisted approaches in 11,500 anatomic lung cancer resections. Ann Thorac Surg 2012;94(2):347–53.
6. Gopaldas RR, Bakaeen FG, Dao TK, et al. Video-assisted thoracoscopic versus open thoracotomy lobectomy in a cohort of 13,619 patients. Ann Thorac Surg 2010;89(5):1563–70.
7. Cerfolio RJ, Bryant AS, Skylizard L, et al. Initial consecutive experience of completely portal robotic pulmonary resection with 4 arms. J Thorac Cardiovasc Surg 2011;142(4):740–6.
8. Dylewski MR, Ohaeto AC, Pereira JF. Pulmonary resection using a total endoscopic robotic video-assisted approach. Semin Thorac Cardiovasc Surg 2011;23(1):36–42.
9. Louie BE, Farivar AS, Aye RW, et al. Early experience with robotic lung resection results in similar operative outcomes and morbidity when compared with matched video-assisted thoracoscopic surgery cases. Ann Thorac Surg 2012;93(5): 1598–605.
10. Park BJ, Flores RM, Rusch VW. Robotic assistance for video-assisted thoracic surgical lobectomy: technique and initial results. J Thorac Cardiovasc Surg 2006;131(1):54–9.
11. Veronesi G, Galetta D, Maisonneuve P, et al. Four-arm robotic lobectomy for the treatment of early-stage lung cancer. J Thorac Cardiovasc Surg 2010;140(1):19–25.
12. Pardolesi A, Park B, Petrella F, et al. Robotic anatomic segmentectomy of the lung: technical aspects and initial results. Ann Thorac Surg 2012; 94(3):929–34.
13. Spaggiari L, Galetta D. Pneumonectomy for lung cancer: a further step in minimally invasive surgery. Ann Thorac Surg 2011;91(3):e45–7.
14. Rodriguez JR. Total portal robotic pneumonectomy. Gen Thorac Cardiovasc Surg 2013;61(9):538–41.
15. Giulianotti PC, Buchs NC, Caravaglios G, et al. Robot-assisted lung resection: outcomes and technical details. Interact Cardiovasc Thorac Surg 2010;11(4):388–92.
16. Roviaro G, Varoli F, Vergani C, et al. Techniques of pneumonectomy. Video-assisted thoracic surgery pneumonectomy. Chest Surg Clin N Am 1999;9(2): 419–36, xi–xii.
17. Conlan AA, Sandor A. Total thoracoscopic pneumonectomy: indications and technical considerations. J Thorac Cardiovasc Surg 2003;126(6): 2083–5.
18. Nwogu CE, Glinianski M, Demmy TL. Minimally invasive pneumonectomy. Ann Thorac Surg 2006;82(1): e3–4.
19. Nwogu CE, Yendamuri S, Demmy TL. Does thoracoscopic pneumonectomy for lung cancer affect survival? Ann Thorac Surg 2010;89(6):S2102–6.
20. Deslauriers J, Grégoire J, Jacques LF, et al. Sleeve lobectomy versus pneumonectomy for lung cancer: a comparative analysis of survival and sites or recurrences. Ann Thorac Surg 2004;77(4):1152–6 [discussion: 1156].

Thoracoscopic Versus Robotic Approaches
Advantages and Disadvantages

Benjamin Wei, MD[a], Thomas A. D'Amico, MD[b],*

KEYWORDS

- Robotic surgery • Video-assisted thoracoscopic surgery • Esophagectomy

KEY POINTS

- Robotic surgery has grown from a nascent technology into what has become a dominant modality for a variety of surgical fields. In general thoracic surgery the use of robotic technology is increasing.
- As the use of robotics proliferates, it will be important to compare it with established thoracoscopic approaches in a systematic fashion, and to continue to evaluate both technologies in terms of short-term outcomes, long-term oncologic efficacy, and cost.
- Robotic technology has several theoretical benefits compared with more widely utilized VATS approaches, but few data exist demonstrating objective clinical superiority.
- Robotic technology adds additional operating room expense compared with equivalent VATS procedures. This is largely as the result of disposable charges (instruments, drapes).

INTRODUCTION

Thoracoscopic surgery was first reported by Christian Jacobaeus, a Swedish internist in the early twentieth century. Jacobaeus used a cystoscope to assist him in the lysis of the intrathoracic adhesions that would occasionally prevent the successful induction of pneumothorax: collapse therapy for cavitary tuberculosis. This practice, which became known as closed intrapleural pneumolysis, was widely used until the advent of streptomycin in 1945 led to pharmacologic treatment of tuberculosis.[1]

Since then, thoracoscopic surgery has undergone a major resurgence. Initially thoracoscopy, or video-assisted thoracoscopic surgery (VATS), was reserved for basic procedures such as pleural biopsy and drainage of effusions, but the procedures performed currently by thoracic surgeons have become increasingly complex. For example, approximately 45% of pulmonary lobectomies in the Society of Thoracic Surgeons General Thoracic Surgery Database are performed thoracoscopically.[2] In addition, VATS is routinely used in the resection of mediastinal tumors, esophagectomy, pneumonectomy, and chest-wall resections.[3]

The benefits of VATS over thoracotomy include shorter length of stay in hospital, decreased pain and narcotic utilization, improved recovery time, and decreased complications including pneumonia and atrial fibrillation.[4,5] In addition, thoracoscopic lobectomy, as opposed to thoracotomy, has been shown to increase the chances that a patient will receive the appropriate adjuvant chemotherapy.[6] Recently, a randomized controlled trial comparing VATS with thoracotomy in esophagectomy for esophageal cancer has also shown benefits in terms of perioperative pulmonary morbidity, hospital stay, quality of life, postoperative pain, and blood loss.[7] In summary, the overall advantages of thoracoscopy over thoracotomy in terms of patient recovery have been fairly well established.

Disclosure: None.
a University of Alabama, Birmingham, AL, USA; b Department of Surgery, Duke University Medical Center, Box 3496, Duke South, White Zone, Room 3589, Durham, NC 27710, USA
* Corresponding author.
E-mail address: thomas.damico@dm.duke.edu

Thorac Surg Clin 24 (2014) 177–188
http://dx.doi.org/10.1016/j.thorsurg.2014.02.001
1547-4127/14/$ – see front matter © 2014 Elsevier Inc. All rights reserved.

The use of robotics, on the other hand, is a newer and less proven modality in the realm of thoracic surgery. Although in some respects an extension of thoracoscopy, in the sense that robotic thoracic surgery allows the surgeon to perform minimally invasive procedures, the use of robotics offers distinct advantages and disadvantages in comparison with VATS. First used in 1985 to perform a neurosurgical biopsy and 3 years later to perform a transurethral resection of the prostate, robotic technology is now used for a variety of complex cardiac, urologic, and gynecologic procedures including mitral valve repair and microsurgical treatment of male infertility.[8,9] The earliest reports of thoracic procedures being done with the assistance of robotics date back to 2002.[10–12] There has been a fairly rapid dissemination of robotic technology in the ensuing decade, with many hospitals in the United States marketing some form of robotic thoracic surgery, despite fairly undefined advantages of the technique. This article addresses the potential benefits and limitations of using the robotic platform for the performance of a variety of thoracic operations.

THORACOSCOPIC VERSUS ROBOTIC THORACIC PROCEDURES
Logistics and Personnel

From the standpoint of planning either a VATS or robotics procedure, familiarity of the operative team with the instruments and setup of the case is critical. At present, the preparation required for performing a robotic thoracic operation is more involved than that for VATS. First, making sure that the robot and console is available for the planned time of the operation is a basic logistical issue that cannot be overlooked. Most hospitals will have only 1 or 2 robots available to their surgeons at any one time, and often require surgeons to prearrange. At present, the only robotic surgery platform being used on patients is the da Vinci Surgical System (Intuitive Surgical; Sunnyvale, CA), which was approved in 2000 by the Food and Drug Administration. This system consists of a 3- or 4-armed robot positioned at the patient's side by the operating table and controlled by a console across the room, away from the sterile area. Coordination with the operating room administrators or, preferably, establishing a set "block time" that ensures robot availability is necessary. The size of the robot and its console(s) may dictate the specific operating room to be used, as certain rooms may be too small to accommodate the equipment and personnel needed. Thoracoscopy, on the other hand, requires only basic video equipment: a scope, a camera, and monitors.

Some hospitals require that the scrub technicians and circulating nurses be credentialed to assist with robotics cases, which adds another level of complexity to arranging these operations. Although this should not understate the desirability of having a dedicated team for VATS cases, there are typically more nurses with adequate training to assist with VATS than with robotics cases.

One disadvantage of robotics is that a skilled assistant, capable of deploying the stapler and performing retraction, is required to be present at the table while the operating surgeon is at the console. This assistant can be a scrub technician, physician assistant, cardiothoracic surgery resident, or even another attending surgeon, depending on the skill required to assist a particular procedure. The assistant, regardless of background, needs to be familiar and comfortable with changing the robotic instruments, troubleshooting port and robotic issues, moving instruments into and out of the thorax safely, passing the stapler around structures that are often vascular in nature, and actively assisting in retraction if necessary. The need for an experienced assistant able to react quickly and effectively to potentially catastrophic bleeding, such as in the case of a ruptured pulmonary artery branch during lobectomy, is a potential disadvantage for the robotic surgeon, who is situated away from the operating table. While communication between team members is critical for any procedure, the challenge in robotic surgery is that nonverbal cues and gestures cannot be conveyed by the surgeon to the rest of team because of their separate locations. In robotics, the surgeon can use the marking software to demonstrate structures and transmit directions to the team on the video screen; during VATS, the surgeon can directly show the assistant what to do with the instruments.

One advantage of robotics is that the surgeon controls the camera, negating the need for a skilled camera operator as is needed during thoracoscopy. On the whole, however, the personnel training, requirements, and codependence in robotic surgery are generally more demanding than those in thoracoscopy.

Positioning, Port Setup, and Camera

Patient positioning is generally similar in thoracoscopic and robotic approaches to the same operation. For robotic cases, the position of the robot in the room relative to the patient should not be overlooked. In general, the surgeon should plan on having the robot approach the patient from the opposite direction of the planned orientation of the instruments. Docking the robot does require additional time, which decreases with experience. One study on robotic thymectomy showed that docking times were reduced from an average of 12.5 minutes to 6 minutes between the first 10 and last 10 thymectomies (P<.001).[13] In terms of ports, robotic operations in the chest use 3 to 4 robotic ports (in addition to the port for the stapler). The da Vinci system accommodates both 5- and 8-mm robotic ports, which are reusable, trocar-based, and made of stainless steel. Current-generation thoracoscopic stapling devices will not fit through the 8-mm port, so they must be deployed either via the additional assistant port or by removing the robotic port and enlarging the incision.

Most thoracoscopic cases use 2 or 3 incisions (2–3 fewer incisions than with robotics) and can be performed with or without commercially available ports. In terms of port placement, robotics surgery requires that ports be triangulated, with the camera in the middle and the working arms on either side. There should be a hand's breadth of distance between the ports to avoid interference between the robotic arms. For some cases, the fourth robotic arm is used to assist with retraction; the port for this retraction arm is placed further away from the camera port than the working arms. Port placement for VATS is more variable between surgeons. Some practitioners of VATS place 3 ports in a triangulated fashion. Others have perfected 2-port or uniportal techniques that do not require triangulation.[14]

The view from the surgeon's console in robotic surgery integrates 2 separate feeds from adjacent camera lenses on the end of the camera, resulting in a 3-dimensional high-definition (HD) image. Although HD systems are readily available for thoracoscopy, the robotic platform reestablishes binocular vision and depth perception that is lost with 2-dimensional thoracoscopy. While the advantage of this degree of visual feedback may seem obvious, whether there is an objective clinical benefit remains untested. Another benefit of the robotic visual system is the magnified view which is particularly helpful in narrow spaces such as the mediastinum. However, this feature can also be a disadvantage when a more global view of the hemithorax is desired.

Instrumentation

A large array of traditional instruments for open thoracic surgery can be used through thoracoscopy incisions, and there is a wide spectrum of dedicated thoracoscopic instruments that are now also available. In contrast there are a limited number of strictly robotic instruments and they have a finite number of uses whereas thoracoscopic instruments are often reusable. Recent advances in robotic instrument technology include a vessel sealer, suction irrigator and stapling devices. Vascular staplers compatible with the robotic system are not yet available.

Robotics instruments currently allow for more degrees of freedom than thoracoscopic instruments, and robotic arms allow a greater variety of angles of approach toward structures in the chest. This wristed maneuverability allows the surgeon to achieve in more complex movements, such as suturing with greater ease. The robot also offers motion scaling: the console translates the surgeon's larger movements to the smaller movements of the instruments commanded inside the body, neutralizing surgeon tremor. From an ergonomic perspective, because the surgeon is seated at the console, fatigue and musculoskeletal issues related to prolonged periods of standing may pose less of an issue, on both an immediate and long-term basis. However, robotic instruments have no haptic feedback to the operating surgeon. Therefore, the surgeon must rely entirely on visual cues for dissection and manipulation of the tissue. Because the robot is capable of transmitting considerable force to tissue, the surgeon must maintain constant vigilance to avoid inadvertent injuries.

Training

The training paradigm for robotic surgeons is beginning to be established. Advantages of training in VATS include its broader applicability, as skills learned during less technically demanding procedures such as wedge resection and decortication can be applied to more complex operations. Although a similar process of moving from simpler to more complex procedures should be undertaken during the training process with robotic surgery, the argument for going back to doing the simpler procedures with the robot is difficult to sustain because of the additional cost and time needed with little apparent advantage to the patient. Having the surgeon and trainee change roles within an operation is more involved in robotic surgery, given that one will be at the operating table and the other at the console. Robotic systems with dual consoles do, however, facilitate having the mentor and trainee operate together in order to learn in a stepwise fashion. Working on simulation programs and operating on cadavers is thought to be necessary before performing robotic thoracic surgery, while not part of the typical VATS teaching model at academic medical centers to date.[15] Because of the widespread usage of VATS, the typical thoracic trainee has extensive exposure to VATS during his or her residency, whereas robotics is still used on a limited basis for thoracic surgery in most medical centers at present.

Opportunities to become proficient in robotics are, therefore, currently more limited. Veronesi and colleagues[16] reported the learning curve for robotic lobectomy to be 18 cases, based on significantly decreased operating time between the first and second terciles of procedures performed. Zhao and colleagues[17] estimated the learning curve for VATS lobectomy to be 30 cases, based on a plateau in operating time and blood loss. The definition of learning curve, however, varies between studies and is affected by how the investigators choose to group cases for analysis. To date there has been no research directly comparing the learning curves between robotics and VATS. Therefore, there exist no objective data on whether robotics or VATS is "easier" to learn.

Cost

The additional costs of robotics in comparison with VATS for lobectomy has been studied by Park and Flores,[18] who estimated that a robotic lobectomy cost an additional US$3981 compared with VATS, $3880 of which was on the day of the operation. Both robotic and VATS lobectomy, however, were significantly less expensive than lobectomy via thoracotomy. Robotic thymectomy was estimated to cost €1701 ($2279) more than VATS thymectomy by an Austrian group.[19] A da Vinci SI robotic surgical system with dual console technology currently costs between $1.3 and $2.2 million in the United States with an annual maintenance cost of approximately $170,000 per year.[20] Use of an individual robotic instrument during a procedure costs approximately $200 ($2000/10 total uses). In 2010, investigators studying 20 types of surgery being performed robotically found that the per-procedure cost of using the robot was approximately an additional $1600, or 6% of the cost of the operation. If the amortized cost of the robot itself was included, this theoretically rose to $3200, or 13% of the cost of the operation.[21] If additional vendors develop robotic surgical platforms and competition increases, the price of the devices may decrease. At present, however, using robotics clearly costs more than VATS for a given procedure.

Telesurgery

The fact that the surgeon operates from the console allows for robotic surgery to be theoretically performed from remote locations (telesurgery), which was demonstrated on the Zeus robotic platform (since discontinued) in the so-called Lindbergh operation, which involved a cholecystectomy performed on a patient in France by a surgeon located in New York.[22] A Canadian group performed 22 telesurgeries, including colectomy, fundoplication, and inguinal hernia repair, from a distance of more than 400 km away, also using the Zeus platform.[23] Robotic telesurgery for thoracic procedures has not yet been reported, but is conceivable.

ROBOTIC VERSUS THORACOSCOPIC THYMECTOMY

Before the advent of thoracoscopy, thymectomy was typically performed via median sternotomy. However, VATS thymectomy has now become an accepted method for resection of the thymus in nonthymomatous myasthenia gravis (MG) and early-stage thymoma (with or without MG). Sternotomy remains the approach of choice for most surgeons in patients with locally invasive thymomas. VATS resection is often used for thymomas less than 5 cm in diameter, but it has also been used successfully for larger tumors. Multiple studies have demonstrated decreased blood loss,[24–26] shorter length of stay in hospital,[24,27,28] and at least equivalent symptomatic outcomes in patients with MG[25,28,29] undergoing VATS thymectomy, compared with transsternal thymectomy.

Proponents of robotic thymectomy argue that working in the anterior mediastinum is inherently awkward and poorly visualized by VATS, and therefore that a complete resection of the thymic horns extending into the superior mediastinum and neck is difficult to accomplish. Given that comprehensiveness of resection has been shown to correlate with an improved response rate in terms of MG symptoms, this assertion has implications for the relative effectiveness of the procedures.[30] Practitioners of VATS thymectomy, on the other hand, believe that they can achieve a complete dissection of the thymus thoracoscopically at low cost and with less complexity than a robotic approach. One unresolved question for VATS thymectomies is whether a unilateral or bilateral approach is more effective and, if unilateral, whether a right-sided or left-sided approach is better. Both bilateral and unilateral VATS thymectomies have been reported with good symptomatic results in MG patients.[24,31] No direct comparisons with regard to superiority of either strategy (unilateral vs bilateral) have been made. Nevertheless, if improved visualization of the thymic tissue and surrounding structures (phrenic nerve, innominate vein) can obviate routine bilateral entry into the chest, this would offer a significant advantage of robotics over VATS.

A prospective, randomized controlled trial of thoracoscopic versus robotic thymectomy has not been performed. Ruckert and colleagues[32] conducted a retrospective cohort study of 79 VATS thymectomies and 74 robotic thymectomies for patients with MG in the largest comparison of the methods to date. The anatomic boundaries of resection were identical in both groups. The approach was unilateral in nature in both the robotic and VATS groups, from the left in nonthymoma patients and from the right in thymoma patients. The visualization between the two groups differed in that carbon dioxide insufflation to a pressure of 5 mm Hg was performed for the robotic thymectomies. The patients in each group were similar in terms of demographics and severity of MG. Operative time was similar (187 ± 48 minutes for robotic compared with 198 ± 48 minutes for VATS). The rate of conversion to sternotomy (1.2% robotic vs 1.3% VATS) and postoperative morbidity rate (2.7% robotic vs 2.5% VATS) were also comparable. The investigators did find a significantly increased complete remission rate of MG at 42 months following resection for the robotic group when compared with the VATS group (39.25% vs 20.3%, $P = .01$). The follow-up was standardized at 42 months for each patient in both groups. The investigators postulated that the difference in results was due to increased completeness of resection, owing to either robotic technology or improved visualization as a result of insufflation. Another possible explanation not mentioned is that the experience gained with VATS thymectomy (done from 1994 to 2002) translated into better outcomes later with robotics (done from 2003 to 2006).

The noncomparative case series in the literature support the safety of robotic thymectomy for both nonthymomatous MG patients and early-stage (I and II) thymomas. Complication rates and median length of stay appear to be comparable with those of VATS thymectomy.[33] Short-term to midterm results of robotic thymectomy for relief of MG symptoms have been reported, but long-term (>10 year) results are unknown. Freeman and colleagues[34] found that improvement in MG symptoms as defined by the Myasthenia Gravis Foundation of America classification occurred in 87% of patients at a mean follow-up time of 45 ± 14 months after robotic thymectomy, with all 75 patients completing the 36-month follow-up visit. Goldstein and Yang[35] reported an 82% improvement in patient symptoms at a mean follow-up of 26 months after robotic thymectomy. A clinical improvement rate of approximately 90% has been reported by 2 other studies of robotic thymectomy (median follow-up 17–24 months).[12,36] These results are comparable with rates obtained in VATS thymectomy for MG patients, which range from 81% to 96%.[37–40] Longer-term (>5 year) MG symptom relief rates are unknown for robotic surgery, while the results for VATS thymectomy are comparable with those for open thymectomy.[37,41,42] For patients with thymomas, only short-term (14–40 months median follow-up) studies have examined the question of recurrence following robotic surgery.[33,43] The chance of recurrence after VATS thymectomy for thymoma, though similar at 5 years in comparison with open thymectomy, is also not well documented at further time points.[27] Given that thymoma recurrence tends to occur 10 to 15 years following the operation, the authors cannot comment meaningfully on the ultimate recurrence risk following either robotic or VATS thymectomy for thymomas at this point.

Robotic and VATS thymectomies are, by and large, similar in terms of potential patient selection, complication rates, hospitalization, and short-term success rates for MG relief and thymoma resection. Because of the relatively recent adoption of both methods (in comparison with resection via sternotomy), there is currently an absence of data on either long-term MG symptom relief or long-term recurrence risk for early-stage thymomas. Thus the advantages of robotics versus VATS for thymectomy at this point seem to be fairly subjective and a matter of technical preference. For the surgeon who is experienced in VATS and can accomplish a true complete resection of thymus, robotics is probably unlikely to yield benefit. However, for practitioners who find the approach to the anterior mediastinum via VATS awkward and the structures in this limited space difficult to visualize and manipulate, robotics may offer a more satisfactory result in terms of extent of resection and, by inference, ultimate outcome.

ROBOTIC VERSUS THORACOSCOPIC PULMONARY RESECTION

Thoracoscopic lobectomy has become a well-established technique in the armament of the modern thoracic surgeon. Experienced practitioners of thoracoscopic lobectomy have demonstrated excellent safety and a conversion rate of 1% to 2%.[44–47] Compared with thoracotomy, thoracoscopic lobectomy offers less postoperative pain, decreased length of hospital stay, and reduced morbidity.[4,48]

In addition, the oncologic outcomes of VATS have been shown to be at least comparable to those of open lobectomy for lung cancer.[49] Investigators have demonstrated that mediastinal lymph node dissection is equivalent whether lobectomy is performed with thoracotomy or thoracoscopy.[50] Recently, however, concerns have been raised that for less-experienced surgeons, mediastinal lymph node dissection is inferior in VATS in comparison with thoracotomy.[51] Although the extent of lymph node dissection in lobectomy has not yet been linked with patient survival, obtaining an adequate lymph node dissection does have implications for the appropriate staging of patients and delivery of adjuvant therapy.[52,53] Some proponents of robotic lobectomy believe that the platform offers them better hilar and mediastinal lymph node dissection as a result of the improved view and more sophisticated articulation of the instruments.

Some practitioners believe that the 3-dimensional optics and the articulation provided by robotic instruments may allow for increased use of a minimally invasive approach to pulmonary resection. The learning curve for robotic prostatectomy has been shown to be similar between fellowship-trained laparoscopic surgeons and experienced practitioners of open prostatectomy.[54] If the learning curve for robotic pulmonary lobectomy were similar, minimally invasive lobectomy might become more accessible to practitioners who are well-versed in open surgery but did not train in the VATS era.

Although there are few published series of robotic lobectomies, and none with the total numbers reported in the largest series of VATS lobectomies, the existing data suggest that robotic lobectomy does offer similar advantages to VATS in terms of postoperative morbidity and recovery, compared with thoracotomy. Cerfolio and colleagues[55] compared a series of 106 patients who underwent robotic lobectomies with 318 matched patients who underwent lobectomy via "rib and nerve-sparing" thoracotomy. The group demonstrated reduced perioperative morbidity (27% vs 38%, $P = .05$), improved mental quality of life (score of 53 vs 40 on the 12-item Short-Form Health Survey, $P<.001$), shorter chest-tube duration (1.5 vs 3 days, $P<.001$), and shorter hospital stay (2 vs 4 days, $P = .02$) in the robotic group. The conversion rate from robotic to open lobectomy was 9%. Park and colleagues[56] reported median length of stay of 5 days, 25% perioperative morbidity, 0.3% mortality, and 8% conversion rate in a multicenter retrospective series of 325 patients undergoing robotic lobectomy for early-stage non–small cell lung cancer. These studies

reported a median operative time of 206 minutes, significantly longer than even the first multi-institutional series on thoracoscopic lobectomy.[57]

Pardolesi and colleagues,[58] in a series of 17 patients who underwent robotic segmentectomy, reported a 0% mortality rate, 17.6% morbidity rate, 5-day median length of stay in hospital, 0% conversion rate, and mean operative time of 189 minutes. These results are comparable with those achieved for VATS segmentectomy.[59]

The only study to date directly comparing robotic and thoracoscopic pulmonary resection was a case-control analysis of anatomic robotic and VATS lung resections: 46 robotic resections (40 lobectomies, 5 segmentectomies, 1 conversion to VATS included in this group for intention-to-treat analysis) were compared with 34 VATS resections (27 lobectomies, 7 segmentectomies).[60] Gender, age, comorbidities, pulmonary function, and American Society of Anesthesiologists status were similar between the two groups; the robotic group, however, had a significantly higher percentage of patients with better performance status (Eastern Cooperative Oncology Group status 0). Parameters such as the size of tumor (median 2.8 cm robotic vs 2.3 cm VATS), operative time (213 minutes robotic vs 207 minutes VATS), length of stay (4.0 days robotic vs 4.5 days VATS), and postoperative major morbidity (17% robotic vs 15% VATS) and minor morbidity (26% robotic vs 21% VATS) were similar between the robotics and VATS groups. The investigators found that the percentage of expected nodal stations sampled was similar between robotic and VATS cases. One surprising conclusion of the study was that the duration of narcotic use was shorter, and return to usual activities/work sooner, for the robotic lobectomy patients than for the VATS patients. The investigators postulated that this might be the result of less injury to the ribs and neurovascular bundle in robotics cases, whereby the hinge point for movement of instruments occurs inside the chest at the articulating "wrist" as opposed to at the chest wall, as in VATS. However, as the investigators themselves note, this was a nonblinded study that did not use formal pain scales or quantify narcotic use.

From the small number of existing studies, it appears that robotic pulmonary resection can be performed in a safe and reasonably expeditious way that is comparable with VATS in terms of postoperative recovery and morbidity. Although some surgeons believe that robotic mediastinal lymph node dissection is improved in comparison with VATS, there are no objective data to support this claim at present. The question of better postoperative pain in robotic as opposed to VATS lung resection, though suggested in one study, also remains unanswered. It is clear that compared with thoracoscopic lobectomy, robotic lobectomy is associated with longer procedure times and higher costs.

ROBOTIC VERSUS THORACOSCOPIC ESOPHAGEAL SURGERY
Antireflux Procedures

Antireflux procedures such as Nissen fundoplication were among the first esophageal operations to be performed with robotic assistance. There have been several randomized controlled trials comparing robotic fundoplication (RF) with laparoscopic fundoplication (LF).[61–66] These randomized studies, along with additional clinical controlled trials,[67–69] were the subject of a meta-analysis in 2009 that encompassed 533 patients (198 undergoing RF vs 335 patients undergoing LF).[70] The investigators concluded that the postoperative complication rate was lower for RF (odds ratio = 0.35, P = .04), but at the expense of 24 minutes longer total operating time. None of the studies analyzed demonstrated a difference in postoperative complications between the two groups. Early postoperative symptom relief, hospital stay, and patient satisfaction were also not different between RF and LF, but the longest follow-up on a randomized trial to date has only been 12 months.[71] One study did show a lower esophageal acid exposure time (EAET) in patients undergoing RF as opposed to LF (0.2% vs 1%, P = .001), and fewer patients with abnormal postoperative EAET times (0% RF vs 14% LF, P = .026).[72] Both groups, however, demonstrated significant reduction in EAET time compared with preoperative values, and the difference between the RF and LF groups on esophageal pH monitoring did not translate into a difference in symptom relief between the two groups. Another nonrandomized study of 40 patients showed a significant decrease in the rate of patients taking antisecretory medication 6 months after antireflux surgery (0% in the RF group vs 30% in the LF group).[73] With the exception of these end points in these 2 studies, however, the improved visualization of the hiatal structures, more facile knot-tying, and greater simplicity of encircling the distal esophagus, all advantages that have been attributed to the robotic platform for fundoplication, have not translated into improved clinical outcome. At present, although there have been some studies suggesting improved acid reduction following RF compared with LF in terms of parameters such as EAET and antisecretory medication use, the data demonstrate that RF offers short-term subjective patient benefits that are similar to those of LF. RF generally has been shown to require longer operative times and greater cost than LF.

Heller Myotomy

The performance of esophagomyotomy for achalasia requires meticulous attention to the depth of myotomy performed so as to avoid perforation. Historically, the rate of iatrogenic perforation has been 5% to 15% in laparoscopic Heller myotomy (LHM).[74] Although no randomized studies have been performed, multiple case series show that robotic Heller myotomy (RHM) results in a minimal risk of iatrogenic perforation. Melvin and colleagues[74] reported 104 patients undergoing RHM with no perforations. Other nonrandomized studies have shown 0% risk of perforation in the RHM group, compared with an 8% to 16% risk in the LHM group.[75–77] There may be an element of selection bias when evaluating the multiple case series in existence (groups experiencing a high perforation rate with RHM would be less likely to publish their results). Moreover, certain groups have demonstrated extremely low (1%–2%) perforation rates with LHM that are comparable with those of RHM, although these appear to be the minority of reports.[78,79] In a multicenter retrospective analysis of 2683 patients undergoing open Heller myotomy, LHM, and RHM, the perioperative morbidity, mortality rate, and length of stay were similar between LHM and RHM groups.[80] There was no comparison between perforation rate between LHM and RHM in this analysis. Although no randomized data exist, RHM does seem to offer a decreased risk of esophageal perforation compared with LHM. Although it has not yet translated into decreased length of stay in hospital or cost when studied on a larger scale, this advantage appears to be a significant one favoring RHM over LHM.

Esophagogastrectomy

Minimally invasive esophagectomy (MIE) with thoracoscopic intrathoracic esophageal mobilization and laparoscopic gastric conduit preparation has been shown to be a safe operation, with excellent perioperative results.[81] There are recent data from a randomized trial to suggest that VATS offers reduced pulmonary complications following esophagogastrectomy in comparison with thoracotomy.[7] Limiting the extent of thoracic incisions with robotics would seem to offer benefits similar to those of MIE. Robotic-assisted esophagectomy (RE) has recently been described, using the robotic platform for both the thoracic and abdominal phases of esophagectomy.[82] The only study to date comparing RE to MIE was a retrospective review of 37 patients (26 patients in the MIE group, 11 patients in the RE group) who underwent 3-incision esophagogastrectomy with the use of robotics limited to the intrathoracic stage of the procedure.[83] The investigators reported no significant differences in operative time, blood loss, number of resected lymph nodes, postoperative complications, or lengths of stay in the intensive care unit and hospital. One limitation of this study was the small sample size, which would be unlikely to show a significant difference between the two groups in outcome. Data remain scarce regarding the oncologic efficacy of both RE and MIE. One study of 47 patients undergoing RE demonstrated a median disease-free survival of 15 months (median follow-up 35 months), although nearly half of the patients had Stage IVA disease.[84] Five-year disease-free survival has been shown to be similar between patients undergoing MIE and open esophagectomy although, just as with RE, longer-term data do not exist for MIE.[85] Therefore, the oncologic efficacy of RE in comparison with MIE is not easily assessed.

The potential benefit of improved lymphadenectomy in esophagectomy as a result of better optics and articulating instruments has not yet been demonstrated. The yield of lymphadenectomy with RE has been variable, ranging from an average of 12 to 38 lymph nodes harvested.[86] Operative time has also ranged widely between studies, much of which reflects the variety of methods of esophagectomy performed. Galvani and colleagues[84] reported a mean operative time of 267 minutes for robot-assisted transhiatal esophagectomy. Cerfolio and colleagues[82] reported a median time of 367 minutes for robot-assisted Ivor-Lewis esophagectomy. Kernstine and colleagues[87] reported a mean operative duration of more than 600 minutes for completely robotic 3-field esophagectomy, although it should be noted that this reflected total operating time as opposed to incision-to-closure time. Based on the available data, however, robotic mobilization of the esophagus appears to take longer than VATS mobilization: a range of 173 to 180 minutes for RE (excluding RE in prone position) versus 90 to 123 minutes for VATS.[88–91] Stapled anastomoses have been associated with an increased risk of anastomotic stricture when compared with hand-sewn anastomoses.[92] This aspect has traditionally been a limitation of VATS Ivor-Lewis esophagectomy, as performing an intracorporeal anastomosis is difficult with VATS. One potential advantage of RE is that it may allow practitioners to perform hand-sewn

esophagogastric anastomoses within the chest on a more routine basis and thereby decrease the stricture rate. One potential disadvantage of RE over MIE may be increased traumatization of the gastric conduit as a result of the lack of haptic feedback on the robotic console, which has led one team to deliver their conduits with laparoscopy.[82]

In summary, the technical advantages of RE over MIE remain hypothetical, although RE appears to be associated with longer intrathoracic mobilization time compared with VATS. The perioperative and short-term results following RE are comparable with those of MIE. Comments regarding the relative oncologic efficacy of RE and MIE are premature at present.

SUMMARY

Over the past decade, robotic surgery has grown from a nascent technology into what has become a dominant modality for complex thoracic operations at several medical centers worldwide. As the use of robotics proliferates, it will be important to compare it with established thoracoscopic approaches in a systematic fashion, and to continue to evaluate both technologies in terms of short-term outcomes, long-term oncologic efficacy, and cost.

REFERENCES

1. Braimbridge MV. The history of thoracoscopic surgery. Ann Thorac Surg 1993;56:610–4.
2. Ceppa DP, Kosinski AS, Berry MF, et al. Thoracoscopic lobectomy has increasing benefit in patients with poor pulmonary function: a Society of Thoracic Surgeons database analysis. Ann Surg 2012;256:487–93.
3. Berry MF, Onaitis MW, Tong BC, et al. Feasibility of hybrid thoracoscopic lobectomy and en bloc chest wall resection. Eur J Cardiothorac Surg 2012;41:888–92.
4. Villamizar NR, Darrabie MD, Burfeind WR, et al. Thoracoscopic lobectomy is associated with lower morbidity compared with thoracotomy. J Thorac Cardiovasc Surg 2009;138:419–25.
5. Paul S, Altorki NK, Sheng S, et al. Thoracoscopic lobectomy is associated with lower morbidity than open lobectomy: a propensity-matched analysis from the STS Database. J Thorac Cardiovasc Surg 2010;139:366–78.
6. Petersen RP, Pham D, Burfeind WR, et al. Thoracoscopic lobectomy facilitates the delivery of chemotherapy after resection for lung cancer. Ann Thorac Surg 2007;83:1245–9.

7. Biere SS, van Berge Henegouwen MI, Mass KW, et al. Minimally invasive versus open oesophagectomy for patients with oesophageal cancer: a multicentre, open-label, randomised controlled trial. Lancet 2012;379:1887–92.

8. Lanfranco AR, Castellanos AE, Desai JP, et al. Robotic surgery: a current perspective. Ann Surg 2004;239:14–21.

9. Parekattil SJ, Cohen MS. Robotic surgery in male infertility and chronic orchialgia. Curr Opin Urol 2010;20:75–9.

10. Melfi FM, Menconi GF, Mariani AM, et al. Early experience with robotic technology for thoracoscopic surgery. Eur J Cardiothorac Surg 2002;21:864–8.

11. Morgan JA, Ginsburg ME, Sonett JR, et al. Advanced thoracoscopic procedures are facilitated by computer-aided robotic technology. Eur J Cardiothorac Surg 2003;23:883–7.

12. Bodner J, Wykpiel H, Wetscher G, et al. First experiences with the da Vinci operating robot in thoracic surgery. Eur J Cardiothorac Surg 2004;25:844–51.

13. Melfi F, Fanucchi O, Davini F, et al. Ten-year experience of mediastinal robotic surgery in a single referral centre. Eur J Cardiothorac Surg 2012;41:847–51.

14. Burfeind WR, D'Amico TA. Thoracoscopic lobectomy. Operat Tech Thorac Cardiovasc Surg 2004;9:98–114.

15. Cerfolio RJ, Bryant AS, Minnich DJ. Starting a robotic program in general thoracic surgery: why, how, and lessons learned. Ann Thorac Surg 2011;91:1729–37.

16. Veronesi G, Galetta D, Maisonneuve P, et al. Four-arm robotic lobectomy for the treatment of early-stage lung cancer. J Thorac Cardiovasc Surg 2010;140:19–25.

17. Zhao H, Bu L, Yang F, et al. Video-assisted thoracoscopic surgery lobectomy for lung cancer: the learning curve. World J Surg 2010;34:2368–72.

18. Park BJ, Flores RM. Cost comparison of robotic, video-assisted thoracic surgery and thoracotomy approaches to pulmonary lobectomy. Thorac Surg Clin 2008;18:297–300.

19. Augustin F, Schmid T, Sieb M, et al. Video-assisted thoracoscopic surgery versus robotic-assisted thoracoscopic surgery thymectomy. Ann Thorac Surg 2008;85:S768–71.

20. Eisenberg A. When robotic surgery leaves just a scratch. New York Times 2012.

21. Brabash GI. New technology and health care costs—the case of robot-assisted surgery. N Engl J Med 2010;363:701–4.

22. Marescaux J, Leroy J, Rubino F, et al. Transcontinental robot-assisted remote telesurgery: feasibility and potential applications. Ann Surg 2002;235:487–92.

23. Anvari M. Remote telepresence surgery: the Canadian experience. Surg Endosc 2007;21:537–41.

24. Jurado J, Javidfar J, Newmark A, et al. Minimally invasive thymectomy and open thymectomy: outcome analysis of 263 patients. Ann Thorac Surg 2012;94:974–81.

25. Lin MW, Chang YL, Huang PM, et al. Thymectomy for non-thymomatous myasthenia gravis: a comparison of surgical methods and analysis of prognostic factors. Eur J Cardiothorac Surg 2010;37:7–12.

26. Shiono H, Kadota Y, Hayashi A, et al. Comparison of outcomes after extended thymectomy for myasthenia gravis: bilateral thoracoscopic approach versus sternotomy. Surg Laparosc Endosc Percutan Tech 2009;19:424–7.

27. Pennathur A, Qureshi I, Schuchert MJ, et al. Comparison of surgical techniques for early-stage thymoma: feasibility of minimally invasive thymectomy and comparison with open resection. J Thorac Cardiovasc Surg 2011;141:694–701.

28. Meyer DM, Herbert MA, Sobhani NC, et al. Comparative clinical outcomes of thymectomy for myasthenia gravis performed by extended transsternal and minimally invasive approaches. Ann Thorac Surg 2009;87:385–90.

29. Bachmann K, Burkhardt D, Schreiter I, et al. Long-term outcome and quality of life after open and thoracoscopic thymectomy for myasthenia gravis: analysis of 131 patients. Surg Endosc 2008;22:2470–7.

30. Zielinski M, Hauer L, Hauer J, et al. Comparison of complete remission rates after 5 year follow-up of three different techniques of thymectomy for myasthenia gravis. Eur J Cardiothorac Surg 2010;37:1137–43.

31. Yu L, Zhang X, Shan M, et al. Thoracoscopic thymectomy for myasthenia gravis with and without thymoma: a single-center experience. Ann Thorac Surg 2012;93:240–4.

32. Ruckert JC, Swierzy M, Ismail M. Comparison of robotic and nonrobotic thoracoscopic thymectomy: a cohort study. J Thorac Cardiovasc Surg 2011;141:673–7.

33. Marulli G, Rea F, Melfi F, et al. Robot-aided thoracoscopic thymectomy for early-stage thymoma: a multicenter European study. J Thorac Cardiovasc Surg 2012;144:1125–32.

34. Freeman RK, Ascioti AJ, Von Woerkom JM, et al. Long-term follow-up after robotic thymectomy for nonthymomatous myasthenia gravis. Ann Thorac Surg 2011;92:1018–23.

35. Goldstein SD, Yang SC. Assessment of robotic thymectomy using the Myasthenia Gravis Foundation of America guidelines. Ann Thorac Surg 2010;89:1080–6.

36. Rea F, Marulli G, Bortolotti L, et al. Experience with the Da Vinci robotic system for thymectomy in patients with myasthenia gravis: report of 33 cases. Ann Thorac Surg 2006;81:455–9.

37. Savcenko M, Wendt GK, Prince SL, et al. Video-assisted thymectomy for myasthenia gravis: an update of a single institution experience. Eur J Cardiothorac Surg 2002;22:978–83.

38. Mineo TC, Pomepeo E, Lerut TE, et al. Thoracoscopic thymectomy in autoimmune myasthenia: result of left-sided approach. Ann Thorac Surg 2000;69:1537–41.

39. Wright GM, Barnett S, Clarke CP. Video-assisted thoracoscopic thymectomy for myasthenia gravis. Intern Med J 2002;32:367–71.

40. Manlulu A, Lee TW, Wan I, et al. Video-assisted thoracic surgery thymectomy for nonthymomatous myasthenia gravis. Chest 2005;128:3454–60.

41. Keating CP, Kong YX, Tay V, et al. VATS thymectomy for nonthymomatous myasthenia gravis: standardized outcome assessment using the myasthenia gravis foundation of America clinical classification. Innovations 2011;6:104–9.

42. Tomulescu V, Ion V, Kosa A, et al. Thoracoscopic thymectomy: mid-term results. Ann Thorac Surg 2006;82:1003–7.

43. Mussi A, Fanucchi O, Davini F, et al. Robotic extended thymectomy for early-stage thymomas. Eur J Cardiothorac Surg 2012;41:e43–7.

44. McKenna RJ, Houck W, Fuller CB. Video-assisted thoracic surgery lobectomy: experience with 1100 cases. Ann Thorac Surg 2006;81:421–6.

45. Onaitis MW, Petersen RP, Balderson SS, et al. Thoracoscopic lobectomy is a safe and versatile procedure. Ann Surg 2006;244:420–5.

46. Cao C, Manganas C, Ang SC, et al. A meta-analysis of unmatched and matched patients comparing video-assisted thoracoscopic lobectomy and conventional open lobectomy. Ann Cardiothorac Surg 2012;1:16–23.

47. Yan TD, Black D, Bannon PG, et al. Systematic review and meta-analysis of randomized and nonrandomized trials on safety and efficacy of video-assisted thoracic surgery lobectomy for early-stage non-small-cell lung cancer. J Clin Oncol 2009;27:2553–62.

48. Whitson BA, Groth SS, Duval SJ, et al. Surgery for early-stage non-small cell lung cancer: a systematic review of the video-assisted thoracoscopic surgery versus thoracotomy approaches to lobectomy. Ann Thorac Surg 2008;86:2008–16.

49. Rueth NM, Andrade RS. Is VATS lobectomy better: perioperatively, biologically, and oncologically? Ann Thorac Surg 2010;89:S2107–11.

50. D'Amico TA, Niland J, Mamet R, et al. Efficacy of mediastinal lymph node dissection during lobectomy for lung cancer by thoracoscopy and thoracotomy. Ann Thorac Surg 2011;92:226–31.

51. Boffa DJ, Dosinski AS, Paul S. Lymph node evaluation by open or video-assisted approaches in 11,500 anatomic lung cancer resections. Ann Thorac Surg 2012;94:347–53.

52. Scott WJ, Allen MS, Darling G, et al. Video-assisted thoracic surgery versus open lobectomy for lung cancer: a secondary analysis of data from the American College of Surgeons Oncology Group Z0030 randomized clinical trial. J Thorac Cardiovasc Surg 2010;139:976–81.

53. Palade E, Passlick B, Osei-Agyemang T, et al. Video-assisted vs open mediastinal lymphadenectomy for Stage I non-small-cell lung cancer: results of a prospective randomized trial. Eur J Cardiothorac Surg 2013;44(2):244–9.

54. Zorn KC, Orvieto MA, Gong EM, et al. Robotic radical prostatectomy learning curve of a fellowship-trained laparoscopic surgeon. J Endourol 2007;21:441–7.

55. Cerfolio RJ, Brayn AS, Skylizard L, et al. Initial consecutive experience of completely portal robotic pulmonary resection with 4 arms. J Thorac Cardiovasc Surg 2011;142:740–6.

56. Park BJ, Melfi F, Mussi A, et al. Robotic lobectomy for non-small cell lung cancer (NSCLC): long-term oncologic results. J Thorac Cardiovasc Surg 2012;143:383–9.

57. Swanson SJ, Herndon JE, D'Amico TA, et al. Video-assisted thoracic surgery (VATS) lobectomy—report of CALGB 39802: a prospective, multi-institutional feasibility study. J Clin Oncol 2007;25:4993–7.

58. Pardolesi A, Park B, Petrella F, et al. Robotic anatomic segmentectomy of the lung: technical aspects and initial results. Ann Thorac Surg 2012;94:929–34.

59. Atkins BZ, Harpole DH, Magnum JH, et al. Pulmonary segmentectomy by thoracoscopy: reduced hospital length of stay with a minimally-invasive approach. Ann Thorac Surg 2007;84:1107–12.

60. Louie BE, Farivar AS, Aye RW, et al. Early experience with robotic lung resection results in similar operative outcomes and morbidity when compared with matched video-assisted thoracoscopic surgery cases. Ann Thorac Surg 2012;93:1598–605.

61. Cadiere GD, Himpens J, Vertruyen M, et al. Evaluation of telesurgical (robotic) Nissen fundoplication. Surg Endosc 2001;15:918–23.

62. Luketich JD, Fernando HC, Buenaventura PO, et al. Results of a randomized trial of HERMES-assisted versus non-HERMES-assisted laparoscopic antireflux surgery. Surg Endosc 2002;16:1264–6.

63. Draaisma WA, Ruurda JP, Scheffer RC, et al. Randomized clinical trial of standard laparoscopic versus robot-assisted laparoscopic Nissen fundoplication for gastro-oesophageal reflux disease. Br J Surg 2006;93:1351–9.

64. Morino M, Pellegrino L, Giaccone C, et al. Randomized clinical trial of robot-assisted versus laparoscopic Nissen fundoplication. Br J Surg 2006;93: 553–8.

65. Nakadi IE, Melot C, Closset J, et al. Evaluation of da Vinci Nissen fundoplication clinical results and cost minimization. World J Surg 2006;30: 1050–4.

66. Muller-Stich BP, Reiter MA, Wente MN, et al. Robot-assisted versus conventional laparoscopic fundoplication: short-term outcome of a pilot randomized controlled trial. Surg Endosc 2007;21: 1800–5.

67. Heemskerk J, van Gemert WG, Greve JW, et al. Robot-assisted versus conventional laparoscopic Nissen fundoplication: a comparative retrospective study on costs and time consumption. Surg Laparosc Endosc Percutan Tech 2007;17: 1–4.

68. Ceccarelli G, Patriti A, Biancafarina A, et al. Intraoperative and postoperative outcome of robot-assisted and traditional laparoscopic Nissen fundoplication. Eur Surg Res 2009;43:198–203.

69. Hartmann J, Menenakos C, Ordermann J, et al. Long-term results of quality of life after standard laparoscopic vs. robot-assisted laparoscopic fundoplications for gastro-oesophageal reflux disease. A comparative clinical trial. Int J Med Robot 2009;5:32–7.

70. Mi J, Kang Y, Chen X, et al. Whether robot-assisted laparoscopic fundoplication is better for gastroesophageal reflux disease in adults: a systematic review and meta-analysis. Surg Endosc 2010;24: 1803–14.

71. Muller-Stich BP, Reiter MA, Mehrabi A, et al. No relevant difference in quality of life and functional outcome at 12 months' follow-up—a randomized controlled trial comparing robot-assisted versus conventional laparoscopic Nissen fundoplication. Langenbecks Arch Surg 2009;394:441–6.

72. Frazzoni M, Conigliaro R, Colli G, et al. Conventional versus robot-assisted laparoscopic Nissen fundoplication: a comparison of postoperative acid reflux parameters. Surg Endosc 2012;26: 1675–81.

73. Melvin WS, Needleman BJ, Krause KR, et al. Computer-enhanced vs standard laparoscopic antireflux surgery. J Gastrointest Surg 2002;6: 11–5.

74. Melvin SW, Dundon JM, Talamini M, et al. Computer-enhanced robotic telesurgery minimizes esophageal perforation during Heller myotomy. Surgery 2005;138:553–9.

75. Huffmanm LC, Pandalai PK, Boulton BJ, et al. Robotic Heller myotomy: a safe operation with higher postoperative quality-of-life indices. Surgery 2007; 142:613–20.

76. Horgan S, Galvani C, Gorodner MV, et al. Robotic-assisted Heller myotomy versus laparoscopic Heller myotomy for the treatment of esophageal achalasia: multicenter study. J Gastrointest Surg 2005;9:1020–9.

77. Iqbal A, Haider M, Desai K, et al. Technique and follow-up of minimally invasive Heller myotomy for achalasia. Surg Endosc 2006;20:394–401.

78. Finley RJ, Clifton JC, Stewart KC, et al. Laparoscopic Heller myotomy improves esophageal emptying and the symptoms of achalasia. Arch Surg 2001;136:892–6.

79. Roller JE, de la Fuente SG, DeMaria EJ, et al. Laparoscopic Heller myotomy using hook electrocautery: a safe, simple, and inexpensive alternative. Surg Endosc 2009;23:602–5.

80. Shaligram A, Unnirevi J, Simorov A, et al. How does the robot affect outcomes? A retrospective review of open, laparoscopic, and robotic Heller myotomy for achalasia. Surg Endosc 2012;26: 1047–50.

81. Luketich JD, Alvelo-Rivera M, Buenaventrua PO, et al. Minimally invasive esophagectomy: outcomes in 222 patients. Ann Surg 2003;238: 486–95.

82. Cerfolio RJ, Bryant AS, Hawn MT. Technical aspects and early results of robotic esophagectomy with chest anastomosis. J Thorac Cardiovasc Surg 2013;145:90–6.

83. Weksler B, Sharma P, Moudgill N, et al. Robot-assisted minimally invasive esophagectomy is equivalent to thoracoscopic minimally invasive esophagectomy. Dis Esophagus 2012;25:403–9.

84. Galvani CA, Gorodner MV, Moser F, et al. Robotically assisted laparoscopic transhiatal esophagectomy. Surg Endosc 2008;22:188–95.

85. Thomson IG, Smithers BM, Gotley DC, et al. Thoracoscopic-assisted esophagectomy for esophageal cancer: analysis of patterns and prognostic factors for recurrence. Ann Surg 2010;252(2): 281–91.

86. Clark J, Sodergren MH, Purkayastha EK, et al. The role of robotic assisted laparoscopy for oesophagogastric oncologic resection; an appraisal of the literature. Dis Esophagus 2011;24:240–50.

87. Kernstine KH, DeArmond DT, Shamoun DM, et al. The first series of completely robotic esophagectomies with three-field lymphadenectomy: initial experience. Surg Endosc 2007;21: 2285–92.

88. Bodner JC, Zitt M, Ott H, et al. Robotic-assisted thoracoscopic surgery (RATS) for benign and malignant esophageal tumors. Ann Thorac Surg 2005;80:1202–6.

89. Boone J, Schipper ME, Moojen WA, et al. Robot-assisted thoracoscopic oesophagectomy for cancer. Br J Surg 2009;96:878–86.

90. Law SY, Fok M, Wei WI, et al. Thoracoscopic esophageal mobilization for pharyngolaryngoesophagectomy. Ann Thorac Surg 2000;70: 418–22.

91. Smithers BM, Gotley DC, McEwan D, et al. Thoracoscopic mobilization of the esophagus. A 6 year experience. Surg Endosc 2001;15: 176–82.

92. Honda M, Kuriyama A, Noma H, et al. Hand-sewn versus mechanical esophagogastric anastomosis after esophagectomy: a systematic review and meta-analysis. Ann Surg 2013;257:238–48.

Robotic Thymectomy for Myasthenia Gravis

Mahmoud Ismail, MD[a], Marc Swierzy, MD[a], Ralph I. Rückert, MD, PhD[b], Jens C. Rückert, MD, PhD[a],*

KEYWORDS

- Robotic thymectomy • Myasthenia gravis • Thymoma

KEY POINTS

- Robotic thymectomy with the da Vinci robotic system is the latest development in the surgery of thymic gland.
- Thymectomy for myasthenia gravis (MG) is best offered to patients with seropositive acetylcholine receptor antibodies and who are seronegative for muscle-specific kinase protein.
- The robotic operation technique is indicated in all patients with myasthenia gravis in association with a resectable thymoma, typically Masaoka-Koga stages I and II.

INTRODUCTION: NATURE OF THE PROBLEM

MG is an autoimmune neuromuscular disease leading to fluctuating weakness and fatigue of different muscle groups.[1] Thymoma is present in 15% of cases with MG.[2] The thymic gland is located in the anterior mediastinum between both right and left phrenic nerves. In some cases, it is located above or below the phrenic nerve. Ectopic thymic tissue can be located at various locations throughout the anterior mediastinum.[3–5] Therefore, the radicality of thymectomy is crucial for tumor resection and complete remission of MG.[6] Thymectomy is most commonly considered a part of the complex treatment of MG and thymoma.[7] Robotic thymectomy is the latest development in the surgery of the thymus gland.[8] This is primarily because it allows for a complete radical thymectomy, which improves the complete remission rate for MG compared with the conventional thoracoscopic technique.[9] The oncologic outcome in terms of overall survival and thymoma-related survival is promising, but a longer follow-up is needed to consider robotic thymectomy a standard approach.[10]

SURGICAL TECHNIQUE
Preoperative Planning

The evaluation of all patients with MG should be done by a neurologist according to the Myasthenia Gravis Foundation of America (MGFA), ideally in a center specialized for MG. The patients should be divided into age groups and the antibody status for acetylcholine receptor and muscle-specific tyrosine kinase should be evaluated. All patients should undergo a contrast-enhanced CT scan of the thoracic cavity to rule out a concomitant thymic mass. In cases of children and contraindication for a CT scan, MRI of the thoracic cavity can be done. Patients with a thymoma should be discussed by a tumor board. Pulmonary function tests and arterial blood gas analyses are required. All patients should have a thorough neurologic evaluation. For patients with moderate to severely symptomatic MG, the need for preoperative intravenous immunoglobulin therapy or plasmapheresis should be determined by a neurologist and coordinated in the immediate preoperative period. In addition to a neurologic evaluation, all patients

The authors have nothing to disclose.
[a] Bereich Thoraxchirurgie, Charité Universitätsmedizin Berlin, Charitéplatz 1, 10117 Berlin, Germany; [b] Klinik für Chirurgie, Franziskus-Krankenhaus Berlin, Akademisches Lehrkrankenhaus der Charité Universitätsmedizin Berlin, Budapester Strasse 15-19, 10787 Berlin, Germany
* Corresponding author.
E-mail address: jens-c.rueckert@charite.de

Thorac Surg Clin 24 (2014) 189–195
http://dx.doi.org/10.1016/j.thorsurg.2014.02.012
1547-4127/14/$ – see front matter © 2014 Elsevier Inc. All rights reserved

have to be checked for operability due to other diseases.

Variations of Robotic Operative Approach: Which Side?

There are variations in the operative approach to thymectomy, with or without the use of the robotic system: transcervical versus transsternal versus video-assisted thorascopic surgery (VATS). Some thoracic surgeons who perform thymectomy by VATS choose a unilateral or a bilateral approach. The proponents of nonrobotic thoracoscopic

thymectomy more frequently use the bilateral approach to be sure about radical resection.[4] Nevertheless, there are enough data for unilateral nonrobotic technique to be adequate for the suitable anatomic configurations.[11] For robotic thymectomy, there seems to be a better mediastinal dissection possible, and therefore more often (most centers) a unilateral technique has been described (**Table 1**).

Thus, those who perform a unilateral VATS approach and those thoracic surgeons who choose a robotic approach have a similar decision: which side? The major points of consideration

Table 1
Literature summary of robotic thymectomy series including more than 20 cases

Author, Year	Country	Study Interval	Total	MG	Thymoma	Approach	Ports	Complete Remission Rate (%)	Thymoma Recurrence Rate (%)
Ismail et al,[8] 2013	Germany	2003–2012	317	273	56	Left	3	57	0
Keijzers et al,[12] 2013	The Netherlands	2004–2012	138	NA	37	Right	3	NA	2.7
Marulli et al,[10] 2013	Italy	2002–2010	100	100	8	Left	3	28.5	0
Freeman et al,[13] 2011	USA	6-y	75	75	Excluded	Left	3	28	NA
Schneiter et al,[14] 2013	Switzerland	2004–2011	58	25	20	Left	3	NA	11.1
Melfi et al,[15] 2012	Italy	2001–2010	39	19	13	Left	3	NA	0
Seong et al,[16] 2014	Korea	2008–2012	37	NA	11	NA	NA	NA	NA
Augustin et al,[17] 2008	Austria	2001–2007	32	32	9	Right	3	NA	0
Cerfolio et al,[18] 2011	USA	2009–2010	30	30	NA	Right	3	NA	NA
Castle & Kernstine,[19] 2008	USA	2002–2008	26	18	1	Right	4–5	NA	NA
Goldstein et al,[20] 2010	USA	2003–2008	26	26	5	Right	4	NA	NA
Tomulescu et al,[21] 2009	Romania	2008–2009	22	22	Excluded	Left	3	NA	NA
Ye et al,[22] 2013	China	2009–2012	21	0	21	Right	3	NA	0

Abbreviation; NA, Not Announced.

include safety of trocar placement and mediastinal dissection, anatomic considerations for the distribution of thymic tissue, and education as well as ergonomic aspects.[8,18,23–25] Although there is rarely a surgical manipulation of the right phrenic nerve necessary, because there is little if any thymic tissue lateral to or beneath the nerve, avoidance of the right phrenic nerve is easier than on the left.[26,27] Not infrequently, mobilization of the left phrenic nerve is necessary to excise suspicious tissue adjacent to the left thymic lobe, which may extend lateral to or under the nerve. Continual awareness and visualization are required to safely complete this dissection without nerve injury; thus, a left-sided approach may have benefit with respect to this issue.

Another modification of the dissection is inevitable in the occasion of the thymic gland having descended totally or partially posterior rather than anterior to the crossing innominate vein.[27] An anatomic study showed slight advantages in the harvest of ectopic thymic tissue from the left versus right side with thoracoscopy.[28] Further arguments for a left-sided robotic approach include the left thymic portion is usually larger, extends to the cardiophrenic area, and more frequently is affected by neoplastic degeneration. The innominate vein runs mainly in the left part of the upper mediastinal area. Also, the aortopulmonary window as a frequent site of ectopic thymic tissue can be reached better or exclusively from the left side.[25]

The arguments for a right-sided approach include better visualization of the venous confluence from the right side by following the vena cava superior, the visualization and dissection of the aortocaval groove, and better ergonomic position to accomplish dissection from inferiorly working cephalad from the right side.[29] Cerfolio and colleagues[18] suggested also that early in a surgeon's learning curve, a right-sided approach may be easier and safer.[9]

Regardless of the approach, the importance of thinking about the anatomic constraints of every case, appropriate robotic surgical training and education, and rigorous credentialing of practitioners having an optimal chance of radical thymectomy cannot be stressed enough.[30]

Preparation and Patient Positioning

The authors' standard surgical approach for robotic thymectomy in the setting of MG without an associated mass is from the left side using a 3-trocar thoracoscopic procedure. In the event that there is a lesion located mainly in the right thymic lobe, a right-sided approach is chosen. If the lesion is large, or to insure radicality, there should be no hesitation to place an extra trocar in the contralateral side. The surgical procedure is performed under general anesthesia with single-lung ventilation. Communication and coordination with an anesthesiologist is critically important. In a majority of cases, the use of depolarizing agents can be avoided altogether to minimize the risk of postoperative myasthenic crisis. If necessary, however, a 1-time dose of a short-acting depolarizing or nondepolarizing agents may be used.

The patient is placed in a supine position on a vacuum mattress with the operating table slightly tilted to the patient's right side. The left arm is positioned below the table level with flexion at the elbow. The operation field is always prepared and draped for a conversion or to an additional trocar from the right side. The 12-mm trocar for the binocular camera is placed in the fourth intercostal space at the left anterior axillary line. A thoracoscopic 10-mm 30° camera is introduced to evaluate the operation field and help position the other two 8-mm trocars. The cranial trocar is introduced in the third intercostal space at the anterior to middle axillary line, whereas the caudal trocar is located in the fifth intercostal space at the midclavicular line. Thus, all 3 trocars are placed exactly along the submammary fold. The special da Vinci trocars are connected with the 3 robotic arms of the table cart. The Harmonic Shears are placed in the upper trocar whereas the Precise Bipolar Forceps in the lower one.

SURGICAL PROCEDURE

Step 1 (**Fig. 1**): The dissection of the thymic gland starts caudally in the middle of the pericardium parallel to the left phrenic nerve. This

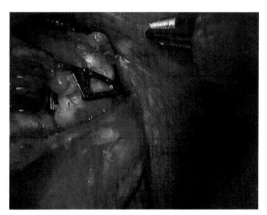

Fig. 1. Dissection of medastinal tissue along the left phrenic nerve. After incision of the mediastinal pleura the phrenic bundle is mobilized.

area is often completely free of fatty tissue, and the left phrenic nerve can be well recognized. But in some cases, the thymic gland extends below or over the phrenic nerve. These cases are optimal for the robotic procedure because it is necessary to isolate the phrenic bundle precisely.

Step 2 (**Fig. 2**): After dissection of the tissue in the aortopulmonary window, further dissection is performed cranially along the phrenic nerve until identifying and opening the cervical pleura at the entrance of the left innominate vein. The incision of the cervical pleural fold is extended to the median retrosternal line. The dissection is continued to the right side until the subxiphoid pleural fold is reached. With blunt gentle dissection, the right lung is made visible and is covered only by the right pleura parietalis. Whenever possible, the right pleural cavity should not be opened to prevent insufflation of CO_2 into the right thoracic cavity (see **Fig. 2**).

Step 3 (**Fig. 3**): The next step is to mobilize and gently pull down the upper poles after careful dissection of their capsule. After that, the thyrothymic ligament becomes clearly visible. Under tension of the completely exposed upper thymic pole, this ligament is severed by ultrasonic dissection or between clip ligatures.

Step 4 (**Fig. 4**): Usually there are 2 to 4 thymic veins that originate from the innominate vein. These veins have to be dissected without tension. The veins are then dissected with ultrasonic scalpel or divided between clip ligatures, depending on the size of the vein and experience of the surgeon. Special attention should be taken for the atypically located thymic veins.

Step 5 (**Fig. 5**): To view the right main thymic lobe, the whole median retrosternal tissue portion has to be mobilized. In most cases, the right main thymic lobe may be demarcated

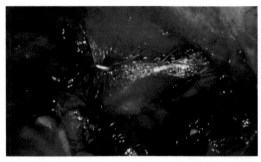

Fig. 3. Mobilization of the left upper thymic pole by gentle dissection and traction with two grasping instruments.

from the surrounding fatty tissue. Also the tissue in the aortocaval groove is dissected free and the right lung, only covered by the mediastinal pleura, is exposed.

Step 6 (**Fig. 6**): Preparation of the right thymic lobe follows mainly under CO_2 insufflation. The right phrenic nerve has to be identified in most cases even before opening the mediastinal pleura of the right lung. The en-bloc resected specimen is placed in a retrieval bag and then removed through the middle trocar incision. The operation field with the venous confluence, the supra-aortic arteries, and parts of the anterior tracheal wall are examined for the presence of residual tissue and hemostasis. A chest tube is placed in the left pleural cavity. Reinflation of both lungs is followed by closure of the trocar incisions.

Immediate Postoperative Care

Patients are extubated immediately postoperatively in the operating room and put on patient-controlled analgesia. Patients can be admitted for 1 night into an ICU or an intermediate care unit. The chest drain is removed if a postoperative chest radiograph shows normal findings during the first 24 hours postoperatively.

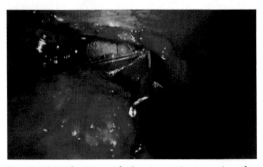

Fig. 2. Identification of the innominate vein after incision of the cervical pleural fold entering the neck area.

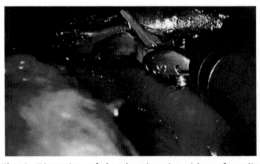

Fig. 4. Dissection of the thymic veins either after clip ligation or ultrasonic dissection.

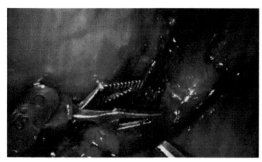

Fig. 5. Deliberation of the right main lobe of the thymic gland from the aorta-caval grove together with the surrounding fatty tissue.

Rehabilitation and Recovery

Patients are normally dismissed between the second and fourth postoperative days after thymectomy. All patients are followed-up by the authors' team, including a neurologist.

CLINICAL RESULTS IN THE LITERATURE

Robotic thymectomy may improve cosmetic results, reduce postoperative pain, and allow accelerated recovery for patients with MG. Worldwide, between 2001 and 2012, there were approximately 3500 robotic thymectomies registered by Intuitive Surgical, Sunny Vale, CA. But the actual number of these operations may be higher and is rising rapidly. **Table 1** lists all published articles with more than 20 robotic thymectomies. Ismail and colleagues[8] described the largest series, containing 317 thymectomies between 2003 and 2012. The main indications were MG and thymoma in 273 and 56 patients, respectively. The operative procedure was performed mainly through a left-sided 3-trocar approach, but for right side–located thymoma, a right-sided approach was chosen. In some cases of large thymoma, a bilateral 3-trocar approach was used. The cumulative complete stable remission rate

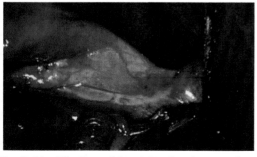

Fig. 6. Identification of the right phrenic nerve from the left side after complete exposure of the venous confluence and the aorto-caval groove.

after robotic thymectomy for MG patients, according to the MGFA postinterventional status, was observed in 57% of the cases. There were no recurrences in patients with thymoma. For limited indications (for instance, in small children, obese patients, and older patients), it seems that robotic thymectomy has a special technical advantage. The actual number of robotic thymectomies in this center from January 2003 to December 2013 is 379.

Keijzers and colleagues[12] reported their 8 years' experience (2004–2012) with robotic thymectomy for thymoma. They retrospectively analyzed the data of 138 robotic procedures for mediastinal tumors and found that the operation indication in 37 patients was for thymoma. The robotic thymectomy was performed through a 3-trocar right-sided approach. The histologic analysis revealed type A (10.8%), type AB (18.9%), type B1 (18.9%), type B2 (37.8%), and type B3 (10.8%) thymomas and thymus carcinoma (2.7%). The Masaoka-Koga stages were as follows: stage I in 20 patients (54%), stage IIA in 5 patients (13.5%), stage IIB in 8 patients (21.6%), stage III in 3 patients (8.1%), and stage IVa in 1 patient (2.7%). There were 5 conversions with 3 R1 resections due to thymus carcinoma or type B2 or B3 thymoma. The median follow-up was 36 months (range 0–79). A recurrence occurred in 1 patient (2.7%) 27 months post-thymectomy (type B2 thymoma, Masaoka-Koga stage IVa). The complete stable remission rate for patients with thymoma and MG was 5%. The investigators conclude that robotic thymectomy is safe in patients with early-stage thymomas and may also be feasible for some selected advanced thymomas.

In a retrospective study, Marulli and colleagues[10] present the results of a series of 100 robotic thymectomies performed between 2002 and 2010. A left-sided 3-trocar procedure was performed. The median patient age was 37 years. Preoperative MGFA class was I in 10% of patients, II in 35% of patients, III in 39% of patients, and IV in 16% of patients. Histologic analysis revealed 76 patients (76%) with hyperplasia, 7 patients (7%) with atrophy, 8 patients (8%) with small thymomas, and 9 patients (9%) with normal thymus. The complete stable remission rate for patients with MG was 28.5%. There were no conversions but in 1 patient a cervicotomy was required to complete dissection of the thymic upper horns. The investigators conclude that robotic thymectomy is a technically sound operation, with low morbidity, short hospitalization, and good neurologic long-term results.

Freeman and colleagues[13] reported on 75 cases of robotic thymectomy over a period of 6 years.

The procedure was performed with a unilateral left-sided 3-trocar technique. The mean age of patients was 38 ± 17 years. There was 1 conversion to sternotomy because of massive pleural adhesions. Histologic classification of resected thymus was normal,[20] involuted,[16] and hyperplastic.[29] The complete stable remission rate for patients with MG was 28%. The investigators conclude that robotic-assisted thymectomy is a safe and effective technique for patients with symptomatic MG. It allowed an extended thymectomy to be performed without the associated length of stay or recovery period of a transsternal approach while producing comparable rates of symptom improvement.

Schneiter and colleagues[14] reported in 2012 about their experience with robotic surgery for anterior mediastinal masses. Of 105 cases, there were 58 patients who underwent robotic thymectomy for thymic disease. The study analyzed the 20 patients with thymoma. The procedure was initially performed as a right-sided 3-trocar technique in the first 15 cases but switched to the unilateral left-sided technique after experience and due to anatomic benefits of the approach. In 5 cases a pericardial resection and in 1 case a lung wedge resection were required. There were no conversions. In 15 patients, a radical robotic thymectomy was performed and in 5 patients with small thymomas a thymomectomy was performed. The investigators reported 3 patients (15%) with R1 resection. The median follow-up time was 26 months (range 0.1–6.6 years). Two patients (11.1%) had a recurrence in the pleura after 1.3 and 4.9 years. One of those patients (5.0%) died because of the recurrence at 5.2 years after surgery. The investigators conclude that robotic thymectomy is save for well-circumscribed thymomas with excellent short- and midterm outcomes.

SUMMARY

Robotic thymectomy is indicated for a majority of patients with MG and early-stage thymoma. The indications have to be discussed by an interdisciplinary board for MG and thymoma. The robotic approach is growing and seems to have a greater potential in terms of technical improvement and outcome as compared to non robotic techniques.

REFERENCES

1. Drachman DB. Myasthenia gravis. N Engl J Med 1994;330(25):1797–810.
2. Papatestas AE, Genkins G, Kornfeld P, et al. Effects of thymectomy in myasthenia gravis. Ann Surg 1987; 206(1):79–88.
3. Masaoka A, Maeda M, Monden Y, et al. Distribution of the thymic tissue in the anterior mediastinum–studies on the methods of thymectomy. Nihon Kyobu Geka Gakkai Zasshi 1975;23(8):1016–21 [in Japanese].
4. Jaretzki A 3rd, Penn AS, Younger DS, et al. "Maximal" thymectomy for myasthenia gravis. Results. J Thorac Cardiovasc Surg 1988;95(5):747–57.
5. Ashour M. Prevalence of ectopic thymic tissue in myasthenia gravis and its clinical significance. J Thorac Cardiovasc Surg 1995;109(4):632–5.
6. Jaretzki A 3rd. Thymectomy for myasthenia gravis. Ann Thorac Surg 1990;49(4):688.
7. Spillane J, Hayward M, Hirsch NP, et al. Thymectomy: role in the treatment of myasthenia gravis. J Neurol 2013;260(7):1798–801.
8. Ismail M, Swierzy M, Ruckert JC. State of the art of robotic thymectomy. World J Surg 2013;37(12): 2740–6.
9. Ruckert JC, Swierzy M, Ismail M. Comparison of robotic and nonrobotic thoracoscopic thymectomy: a cohort study. J Thorac Cardiovasc Surg 2011; 141(3):673–7.
10. Marulli G, Schiavon M, Perissinotto E, et al. Surgical and neurologic outcomes after robotic thymectomy in 100 consecutive patients with myasthenia gravis. J Thorac Cardiovasc Surg 2013;145(3):730–5 [discussion: 5–6].
11. Tomulescu V, Popescu I. Unilateral extended thoracoscopic thymectomy for nontumoral myasthenia gravis–a new standard. Semin Thorac Cardiovasc Surg 2012;24(2):115–22.
12. Keijzers M, Dingemans AM, Blaauwgeers H, et al. 8 Years' experience with robotic thymectomy for thymomas. Surg Endosc 2013. [Epub ahead of print].
13. Freeman RK, Ascioti AJ, Van Woerkom JM, et al. Long-term follow-up after robotic thymectomy for nonthymomatous myasthenia gravis. Ann Thorac Surg 2011;92(3):1018–22 [discussion: 22–3].
14. Schneiter D, Tomaszek S, Kestenholz P, et al. Minimally invasive resection of thymomas with the da Vinci(R) Surgical System. Eur J Cardiothorac Surg 2013;43(2):288–92.
15. Melfi F, Fanucchi O, Davini F, et al. Ten-year experience of mediastinal robotic surgery in a single referral centre. Eur J Cardiothorac Surg 2012; 41(4):847–51.
16. Seong YW, Kang CH, Choi JW, et al. Early clinical outcomes of robot-assisted surgery for anterior mediastinal mass: its superiority over a conventional sternotomy approach evaluated by propensity score matching. Eur J Cardiothorac Surg 2014;45(3):e68–73.
17. Augustin F, Schmid T, Sieb M, et al. Video-assisted thoracoscopic surgery versus robotic-assisted thoracoscopic surgery thymectomy. Ann Thorac Surg 2008;85(2):S768–71.

18. Cerfolio RJ, Bryant AS, Minnich DJ. Starting a robotic program in general thoracic surgery: why, how, and lessons learned. Ann Thorac Surg 2011; 91(6):1729–36 [discussion: 36–7].

19. Castle SL, Kernstine KH. Robotic-assisted thymectomy. Semin Thorac Cardiovasc Surg 2008;20(4): 326–31.

20. Goldstein SD, Yang SC. Assessment of robotic thymectomy using the Myasthenia Gravis Foundation of America Guidelines. Ann Thorac Surg 2010; 89(4):1080–5 [discussion: 5–6].

21. Tomulescu V, Stanciulea O, Balescu I, et al. First year experience of robotic-assisted laparoscopic surgery with 153 cases in a general surgery department: indications, technique and results. Chirurgia (Bucur) 2009;104(2):141–50.

22. Ye B, Tantai JC, Li W, et al. Video-assisted thoracoscopic surgery versus robotic-assisted thoracoscopic surgery in the surgical treatment of Masaoka stage I thymoma. World J Surg Oncol 2013;11:157. http://dx.doi.org/10.1186/1477-7819-11-157.

23. Mulder DG, Graves M, Herrmann C. Thymectomy for myasthenia gravis: recent observations and comparisons with past experience. Ann Thorac Surg 1989;48(4):551–5.

24. Mack MJ. Video-assisted thoracoscopy thymectomy for myasthenia gravis. Chest Surg Clin N Am 2001; 11(2):389–405, xi–xii.

25. Mineo TC, Pompeo E, Ambrogi V. Video-assisted thoracoscopic thymectomy: from the right or from the left? J Thorac Cardiovasc Surg 1997;114(3):516–7.

26. Mulder DG, White K, Herrmann C Jr. Thymectomy. Surgical procedure for myasthenia gravis. AORN J 1986;43(3):640–6.

27. Mulder DG. Extended transsternal thymectomy. Chest Surg Clin N Am 1996;6(1):95–105.

28. Ruckert JC, Czyzewski D, Pest S, et al. Radicality of thoracoscopic thymectomy–an anatomical study. Eur J Cardiothorac Surg 2000;18(6):735–6.

29. Mack MJ, Landreneau RJ, Yim AP, et al. Results of video-assisted thymectomy in patients with myasthenia gravis. J Thorac Cardiovasc Surg 1996; 112(5):1352–9 [discussion: 1359–60].

30. Marulli G, Rea F, Melfi F, et al. Robot-aided thoracoscopic thymectomy for early-stage thymoma: a multicenter European study. J Thorac Cardiovasc Surg 2012;144(5):1125–30.

Robotic Thymectomy for Thymic Neoplasms

Gary S. Schwartz, MD, Stephen C. Yang, MD*

KEYWORDS

- Thymectomy • Thymoma • Robotic

KEY POINTS

- Robotic thymectomy is a minimally invasive technique for removal of thymic tumors.
- A variety of options exist for access, port placement, and specimen retrieval.
- Favorable short- and long-term safety and efficacy of robotic thymectomy for thymic neoplasms have been well demonstrated.

INTRODUCTION

Thymectomy was first reported for the treatment of myasthenia gravis (MG) in 1939.[1] Although the indications for thymectomy—MG and thymoma—have not changed, the surgical technique has evolved significantly. The historical access via a median sternotomy has given way to more minimally invasive techniques, including the transcervical and thoracoscopic approaches.[2] Videoscopic thymectomy can be further enhanced with the aid of a surgical robot. This article provides an overview of the indications, technique, and outcomes of robotic thymectomy for the treatment of thymic masses.

Thymic masses vary in size, gross and microscopic invasion, and histology. They are classified according to the Masaoka-Koga and World Health Organization classification schemes.[3–5] Size is generally accepted as a determinant of operative approach, although no universal guidelines exist. In general, most surgeons agree that lesions 3 cm or less are amenable to minimally invasive approaches because of visualization reasons and the ability to remove them through the small port sites. Case reports have published involving larger tumors, but long-term follow-up on locoregional control and oncologic efficacy are lacking. It is advisable that surgeons who are just beginning

to perform a robotic approach to mediastinal tumors should start with smaller tumors.

Several operative approaches for thymectomy have been described.[6] Traditional thymectomy is performed via a transsternal approach with division of the sternum; however, this approach is accompanied by significant morbidity in 4% to 22% of cases.[7] Additionally, patients with symptomatic MG often have impairment in respiratory function at baseline and inhibition in wound healing because of immunosuppressive medications. For these reasons, minimally invasive approaches to thymectomy have been developed.

Established minimally invasive surgical approaches include transcervical[8] and transthoracic videoscopic thymectomy.[9] These approaches offer radical resection of the thymus with potentially lower morbidity and shorter length of hospital stay compared with open surgical resection via sternotomy. Transcervical thymectomy is limited by size and patients are still at risk for pneumothorax and vascular injuries despite the cervical approach.[10] Some authors propose a combined transcervical and transthoracic approach to ensure completeness of resection.[11]

The thoracoscopic approach can be further optimized with the aid of the da Vinci robotic surgical system (Intuitive Surgical, Mountain View, CA, USA). Robotic-assisted surgery has been

The authors have noting to disclose.

The Johns Hopkins Hospital, 600 North Wolfe Street, Baltimore, MD 21287, USA

* Corresponding author.

E-mail address: syang7@jhmi.edu

Thorac Surg Clin 24 (2014) 197–201

http://dx.doi.org/10.1016/j.thorsurg.2014.02.005
1547-4127/14/$ – see front matter © 2014 Elsevier Inc. All rights reserved.

shown to be safe and feasible in a variety of cardiac, otolaryngologic, gynecologic, and abdominal surgical procedures. The application to thoracic surgery is intuitive, wherein precision of dissection is mandatory but the working space is small and limited by the rigid confines of the chest wall. Resection of anterior mediastinal masses, specifically thymectomy, is an ideal operation to be performed thoracoscopically with the aid of the da Vinci robot. Precision of dissection is mandatory not only because of the vital nature of the structures being dissected but also to avoid overmanipulation of a thymic mass and potential seeding of the mediastinum.

Robotic thymomectomy was first described in 2001,[12] and description of a complete thymectomy using a robotic thoracoscopic approach soon followed in 2003.[13,14] To date, several moderate-sized retrospective series review the international experience with this procedure for MG and thymic malignancies.[15–23] Several different techniques have been described for robotic thymectomies and vary according to different parts of the operation. These components are listed in (**Box 1**).

SURGICAL TECHNIQUE
Preoperative Planning

Patients referred for thymectomy have generally already undergone imaging with either computed tomography (CT) scan or magnetic resonance imaging (MRI). Radiographic characteristics that must be assessed include size, heterogeneity, and presence of infiltration of adjacent structures. Intravenous contrast for the CT scan via the left arm is useful in identifying the proximity of the tumor to the innominate and superior vena cava, and the great vessels. Although no specific size limit exists for performing robotic/video-assisted thoracoscopic surgery (VATS) versus open resection, tumors greater than 3 cm should be

---

Box 1
Components of robotic thymectomies

Single lung isolation versus carbon dioxide (CO_2) insufflation

Patient positioning and padding

Robot console/monitor/arm placement

Right versus left side approach

Length, placement, and number of surgical incisions

Bilateral approach

Extent of resection

Optional neck incision

---

approached by experienced robotic surgeons. Moreover, while invasion of adjacent structures, such as the pericardium or lung does not preclude a minimally invasive approach, these cases should be chosen carefully in order to maintain oncologic efficacy first and foremost.

Preparation and Patient Positioning

An epidural catheter is placed preoperatively for postoperative pain control. General endotracheal anesthesia is induced. Double-lumen intubation with bronchoscopic confirmation is performed; alternatively, some surgeons prefer insufflations of the hemithorax with CO_2 rather than endotracheal lung isolation. If both pleura are used for dissection, then separate lung isolation would be ideal. Radial arterial line monitoring, large-bore venous access, urinary catheterization, and sequential compression devices are institution-dependent. The patient is placed supine with both arms tucked, slightly flexing the right arm to allow more access to the lateral chest. Padding is carefully placed to avoid any pressure points on the face, arms, and legs. The operating table is rotated leftward for a shoulder axis of 30° to the horizontal. The patient is prepared and draped in standard fashion, exposing the entire sternum and chest wall. Hybrid modifications have been added that require access to the contralateral chest.

Surgical Approach

The initial transthoracic approach reported was generally bilateral to ensure complete resection and visualization of the bilateral phrenic nerves.[2] Although bilateral access is still preferred by some surgeons, others maintain that a left-sided approach is superior because of the size differential of the left versus right inferior horn, and proponents of a right-sided approach prefer the additional working space. If the contralateral phrenic nerve is incompletely visualized or aberrant thymic tissue is suspected, bilateral access is mandatory to ensure a radical resection. In the presence of a dominant mass, the ipsilateral side is favored. If neither side is indicated by presence of an ipsilateral mass, the authors favor, an initial unilateral right-sided approach because of the increased working space.[2]

General Preparation

After satisfactory induction of general anesthesia, a double-lumen endotracheal tube or bronchial blocker is correctly placed and positioned. A shoulder roll is placed, and both arms carefully tucked and protected at the patient's sides. Just in case a sternotomy or upper sternal split is needed emergently, the midline is marked at the sternal notch, Louis angle, and xiphoid, because the skin will be distorted once the patient is finally positioned.

Because a right-sided approach is favored by the authors whenever feasible, a small bump is also inserted behind the right chest laterally. The entire table is rotated counterclockwise to the 10 o'clock position for the anesthesiologist, which facilitates positioning of the robot when it is ready to be positioned and docked. The table is then turned steeply to the left, with the hip taped and a padded sled placed on the left side of the bed so the patient and table foam will not slide. In addition, a large square foam pad is taped to the left side of the patient's face to keep the head aligned straight with the body and prevent any injury to the face once the robotic arms are in position and engaged. Obviously, if a left-sided robotic approach is performed, the opposite positioning steps are carried out.

Surgical Procedure

Step 1: port placement
The first port is placed in the anterior axillary line in the fifth intercostal space to allow for initial exploration with a 30° thoracoscope or the robotic camera (**Fig. 1**, camera). Evidence of extensive pleural studding or invasive disease should prompt reconsideration of surgical approach. Three additional ports are placed under direct thoracoscopic vision: left and right arm ports in the third and eighth intercostal spaces (see **Fig. 1**, dissector 1 and cautery, respectively) along the midclavicular line, and a working port/second left arm in the fifth or sixth intercostal space along the midaxillary line (see **Fig. 1**, dissector 2). The robot is then docked

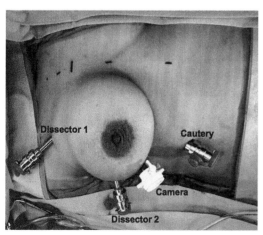

Fig. 1. From cranial to caudal, robotic ports are arranged as follows: dissector 1 (arm 2), dissector 2 (arm 3), endoscope (camera arm), cautery (arm 1).

from the patient's left side over the left shoulder and the instruments loaded. The authors prefer Cardiere forceps in the left 2 working hands and the spatula dissector in the right, although these instruments can be adapted to the surgeon and patient.

Step 2: dissection
The mediastinal pleura is incised and the thymus is mobilized off the anterior mediastinal fat, with care taken to continuously visualize and protect the right phrenic nerve. To minimize potential thermal injury to the phrenic nerve, either bipolar or other low electrothermal energy devices are used to mobilize the mediastinal tissues away. The dissection continues up to the thoracic inlet to the apex of the right cervical horn. Along this plane, thymic veins draining into the innominate vein are encountered and clipped. Dissection is then carried across the midline by dissecting the gland off the posterior shelf of the sternum and advancing toward the left cervical horn. As this is dissected, the use of cautery is minimized until the left phrenic nerve is identified, which can be aided using downward traction on the pericardium. Difficult or incomplete visualization of the nerve should prompt consideration of placement of a left-sided 5-mm port and thoracoscope to aid in visualization. The Si model of the da Vinci robot further enables this exposure with its picture-in-picture feature, allowing the operating surgeon to visualize the thymus and any tumor mass from both perspectives simultaneously. If the dissection cannot be safely completed from the right side, the right lung is reinflated and the dissection is moved to the left chest. Additional ports are placed in a symmetric fashion to the right-sided incisions and the robot is repositioned to allow for dissection to continue from the left chest.

Step 3: specimen retrieval and closure
Once the specimen is completely resected, it is placed in a specimen bag and removed. Depending on the size of the tumor, the camera port is enlarged. The ribs might be gently separated to allow specimen retrieval. Others have described retrieval of larger tumors through a separate incision in the diaphragm and extracted through an abdominal incision.

Pleural drainage tubes are placed according to the operating surgeon's preference; the authors prefer a single 19 French Blake drain through the most inferior port site and guided to the apex along the posterior sulcus and looping around to the anterior mediastinum. The lung is reinflated under direct vision. Skin incisions are closed and dressed in a standard manner.

Immediate Postoperative Care

Patients are extubated in the operating room; otherwise healthy patients recover in the postanesthesia care unit and then the floor, whereas those with significant comorbidities are transferred to the intensive care unit. The pleural tube is placed with gravity drainage overnight and typically removed on postoperative day 1. Patients are discharged home on postoperative day 1 or 2, with follow-up at 2 weeks.

REASONS FOR CONVERTING TO OPEN APPROACH

In general, more than 90% of benign thymic tumors can be resected robotically. Localized invasion into the lung, pericardium, pleura, or diaphragm can still be resected without conversion to open approaches. More difficult situations that may require more aggressive intervention are when the tumor involves major vascular structures and/or the chest wall. In rare situations, uncontrollable bleeding may also need an open approach to achieve hemostasis.

CLINICAL RESULTS IN THE LITERATURE

Outcomes after robotic thymectomy have been reported in a variety of manners. Clinical results have been described in several retrospective reviews of single-center experiences,[15–23] not necessarily differentiating between thymectomy for MG and thymectomy for mediastinal masses. Long-term follow-up varies, with the longest reported period being an average of almost 4 years. Reported outcomes of robotic thymectomy for the treatment of MG have included improvement in remission.[9,19,20,23]

Single-center comparisons of transsternal, VATS, and robotic thymectomy have also been reported. In general, no significant difference in clinical outcome has been observed, with a shorter length of stay and perhaps a more rapidly improved quality of life associated with the robotic approach.[9,11,24] The cost differential is institution-dependent, but the robotic approach can cost as much as 91% more than a VATS approach because of instrument costs and operating room expenses.[21]

Complication rates after robotic thymectomy are comparable to those associated with a VATS approach, with the primary offenders being vascular injury and incomplete resection requiring reoperation.[15–23] Rates of these complications are significantly lower than with the transsternal approach. Additional complications, such as intercostal neuralgia and brachial plexus injury, are also associated with the robotic approach.[25] Length of stay is longer than with a transcervical approach[8]; however, larger glands and masses can be removed and a complete resection is more readily apparent. Additionally, training surgeons in robotic thymectomy seems to be easier than training them in the transcervical approach, wherein visibility is limited to the operating surgeon.[10] Finally, both the VATS and robotic approaches require double-lumen intubation and postoperative pleural drainage, which are not necessary with a transcervical approach.

SUMMARY

The enhanced dexterity and visualization provided by the da Vinci robot is ideal for application to general thoracic surgery, wherein working angles are difficult and vital structures exist in a confined space. As instrumentation and visualization of the robotic approach improve, so will its application to thymectomy. Adaptations of the current transthoracic technique, including a subxiphoid approach,[26] may become feasible, potentially further decreasing the length of stay and complication rate associated with the current technique while ensuring complete resection and maximal improvement in quality of life.

REFERENCES

1. Blalock A, Mason MF, Morgan HJ, et al. Myasthenia gravis and tumors of the thymic region: report of a case in which the tumor was removed. Ann Surg 1939;110:544–61.
2. Yim AP, Kay RL, Ho JK. Video-assisted thoracoscopic thymectomy for myasthenia gravis. Chest 1995;108(5):1440–3.
3. Masaoka A, Monden Y, Nakahara K, et al. Follow-up study of thymomas with special reference to their clinical stages. Cancer 1981;48:2485–92.
4. Koga K, Matsuno Y, Noguchi M, et al. A review of 79 thymomas: modification of staging system and reappraisal of conventional division into invasive and non-invasive thymoma. Pathol Int 1994;44:359–67.
5. Travis WD, Brambilla E, Muller-Hermelink H, et al. Pathology and genetics of tumors of the lung, pleura, thymus and heart. In: Kleihues P, Sobin L, editors. WHO classification of tumors. 2nd edition. Lyon (France): IARC Press; 2004. p. 145–97.
6. Magee MJ, Mack MJ. Surgical approaches to the thymus in patients with myasthenia gravis. Thorac Surg Clin 2009;19(1):83–9, vii.
7. Kas J, Kiss D, Simon V, et al. Decade-long experience with surgical therapy of myasthenia gravis: early complications of 324 transsternal thymectomies. Ann Thorac Surg 2001;72:1691–7.

8. Shrager JB. Extended transcervical thymectomy: the ultimate minimally invasive approach. Ann Thorac Surg 2010;89(6):S2128–34.

9. Meyer DM, Herbert MA, Sobhani NC, et al. Comparative clinical outcomes of thymectomy for myasthenia gravis performed by extended transsternal and minimally invasive approaches. Ann Thorac Surg 2009;87(2):385–90.

10. Calhoun RF, Ritter JH, Guthrie TJ, et al. Results of transcervical thymectomy for myasthenia gravis in 100 consecutive patients. Ann Surg 1999;230(4): 555–9.

11. Rückert JC, Swierzy M, Ismail M. Comparison of robotic and nonrobotic thoracoscopic thymectomy: a cohort study. J Thorac Cardiovasc Surg 2011; 141(3):673–7.

12. Yoshino I, Hashizume M, Shimada M, et al. Thoracoscopic thymomectomy with the da Vinci computer-enhanced surgical system. J Thorac Cardiovasc Surg 2001;122(4):783–5.

13. Ashton RC Jr, McGinnis KM, Connery CP, et al. Totally endoscopic robotic thymectomy for myasthenia gravis. Ann Thorac Surg 2003;75(2):569–71.

14. Bodner J, Cykypiel H, Schmid T. Early experience with robot assisted surgery for mediastinal masses. Ann Thorac Surg 2004;78(1):259–65.

15. Mantegazza R, Baggi F, Bernasconi P, et al. Video-assisted thoracoscopic extended thymectomy and extended transsternal thymectomy (T-3b) in non-thymomatous myasthenia gravis patients: remission after 6 years of follow-up. J Neurol Sci 2003;212: 31–6.

16. Bodner J, Augustin F, Wykypiel H, et al. The da Vinci robotic system for general surgical applications: a critical interim appraisal. Swiss Med Wkly 2005; 135:674–8.

17. Savitt MA, Gao G, Furnary AP, et al. Application of robotic-assisted techniques to the surgical evaluation and treatment of the anterior mediastinum. Ann Thorac Surg 2005;79:450–5.

18. Augustin F, Schmid T, Bodner J. The robotic approach for mediastinal lesions. Int J Med Robot 2006;3:262–70.

19. Rea F, Marulli G, Bortolotti L, et al. Experience with the "da Vinci" robotic system for thymectomy in patients with myasthenia gravis: report of 33 cases. Ann Thorac Surg 2006;81(2):455–9.

20. Cakar F, Werner P, Augustin F, et al. A comparison of outcomes after robotic open extended thymectomy for myasthenia gravis. Eur J Cardiothorac Surg 2007;31(3):501–4.

21. Augustin F, Schmid T, Sieb M, et al. Video-assisted thoracoscopic surgery versus robotic-assisted thoracoscopic surgery thymectomy. Ann Thorac Surg 2008;85(2):S768–71.

22. Freeman RK, Ascioti AJ, van Woerkom JM, et al. Long-term follow-up after robotic thymectomy for nonthymomatous myasthenia gravis. Ann Thorac Surg 2011;92(3):1018–22.

23. Goldstein SD, Yang SC. Assessment of robotic thymectomy using the Myasthenia Gravis Foundation of America Guidelines. Ann Thorac Surg 2010; 89(4):1080–5.

24. Balduyck B, Hendriks JM, Lauwers P, et al. Quality of life after anterior mediastinal mass resection: a prospective study comparing open with robotic-assisted thoracoscopic resection. Eur J Cardiothorac Surg 2011;39(4):543–8.

25. Pandey R, Elakkumanan LB, Garg R, et al. Brachial plexus injury after robotic-assisted thoracoscopic thymectomy. J Cardiothorac Vasc Anesth 2009; 23(4):584–6.

26. Bakker PF, Budde RP, Gründeman PF. Endoscopic robot-assisted extended thymectomy by subxiphoid approach with sternal lifting: feasibility in the pig. Surg Endosc 2004;18(6):986–9.

Robotic Esophagectomy
Modified McKeown Approach

David Lehenbauer, MD, Kemp H. Kernstine, MD, PhD*

KEYWORDS

- Esophageal cancer • Robotics • Minimally invasive surgery • Esophagectomy

KEY POINTS

- Robotic esophagectomy for esophageal carcinoma offers excellent visibility, complex maneuvers, and unprecedented precision during minimally invasive esophagectomy and may ultimately lead to improved outcomes for this difficult disease with profound mortality.
- Further advances in robotics and clinical management comparing robotic resection versus traditional approaches are needed to define the role of robotics in the surgical management of esophageal cancer.

INTRODUCTION

Esophageal carcinoma is a highly lethal disease; untreated, over 95% of symptomatic patients die in less than 12 to 14 months. The incidence of esophageal adenocarcinoma of the esophagus in the United States has demonstrated startling growth in recent years: from 3.6 cases per million population in 1973 to 25.6 cases per million population in 2006.[1] Increases in adenocarcinoma incidence are in part due to growth of the known risk factors gastroesophageal reflux disease and obesity. However, the incidence of squamous cell carcinoma of the esophagus has been steadily decreasing in the western world because of long-term reductions in tobacco abuse and excessive alcohol consumption.

Cure is the ultimate goal for surgical management of esophageal carcinoma. For early stage disease, less than T2, surgery alone has been shown to provide survival benefit as well as prognostic information. For patients with locally advanced disease, 2 randomized trials comparing chemoradiotherapy alone to chemoradiotherapy followed by surgery have failed to demonstrate improved survival with surgery; however, both showed better locoregional control and a lesser need for palliative procedures when surgery was a component of treatment.[2,3] Surgically-related mortality was excessive, diluting the true impact of surgical resection. More recent randomized trials have demonstrated survival benefit, especially in patients resected by means of an optimal minimally invasive approach. Therefore, surgery remains the preferred treatment approach for clinically resectable esophageal cancer.

Esophagectomy is a technically challenging operation. Open esophagectomy has been documented to be effective in providing good oncologic control but often is associated with significant morbidity and postoperative hospital stay. Minimally invasive esophagectomy offers several advantages over the traditional open approach: fewer postoperative complications, less intraoperative blood loss, smaller incisions, shorter hospital and intensive care unit stays, and better preservation of postoperative pulmonary function.[4,5] The surgical optimal approach, open technique versus laparoscopic/thoracoscopic; modified McKeown versus Ivor Lewis versus transhiatal; and various different resection techniques have yet to be determined as to effectiveness. Criticism of minimally invasive esophagectomy has included the uncertainty of adequate lymph node dissection

The authors have nothing to disclose.
Department of Cardiothoracic and Vascular Surgery, University of Texas Southwestern, 5323 Harry Hines Boulevard, HA9.134, Dallas, TX 75390-8879, USA
* Corresponding author.
E-mail address: kemp.kernstine@utsouthwestern.edu

Thorac Surg Clin 24 (2014) 203–209
http://dx.doi.org/10.1016/j.thorsurg.2014.02.002
1547-4127/14/$ – see front matter © 2014 Elsevier Inc. All rights reserved.

and the steep learning curve for mastering the procedure. The computer-assisted technology of the robotic approach to the minimally invasive esophagectomy has the potential to increase lymph node dissection in difficult-to-reach areas and shorten the learning curve. This article will review the technical aspects of the modified McKeown approach to robotic esophagectomy and review the existing literature with respect to indications and outcomes.

SURGICAL TECHNIQUE
Preoperative Planning

Standard workup of esophageal cancers and esophagogastric junction cancers is described by NCCN Clinical Practice Guidelines In Oncology (NCCN Guidelines®) and is shown in **Table 1**.

Patients with T1 or T2 lesions without evidence of nodal disease or metastasis are candidates for esophagectomy as the initial therapeutic approach. Patients with full-thickness lesions or invasion of local structures even with evidence of nodal disease may be candidates for esophagectomy following response to chemotherapy or chemoradiotherapy. The relative contraindication for esophagectomy with advanced age is severe comorbid illness. The presence of lung, bone, adrenal, brain, liver, or peritoneal metastasis precludes resectability. Celiac, mediastinal, and supraclavicular nodes are considered regional nodal disease in the 2010 update for the TNM staging system.

Utilization of robot assistance for esophagectomy requires additional preoperative preparation. Robotic surgery can be performed in patients with history of prior thoracic surgery, but extensive pleural adhesions may preclude a reasonable dissection. Preoperative computed tomography (CT) is beneficial to determine operability and for planning port placement. Generally, port placement should be at least 10 to 15 cm away from pathology, a challenge for small adults and children.

Pulmonary function testing and preoperative cardiac testing will determine if the patient is physiologically fit to undergo esophagectomy. Preoperative evaluation will need to demonstrate that the patient will tolerate CO_2 insufflation and single lung ventilation. A retrospective cohort study demonstrated that patients undergoing an esophagectomy had fewer postoperative complications (6% vs 24%) with preoperative respiratory rehabilitation.[6]

PREPARATION AND PATIENT POSITIONING
Thoracic Phase

At the outset of the procedure, the patient is intubated with a double-lumen endotracheal tube,

---

Table 1
NCCN Guidelines® for Esophageal and Esophagogastric Junction Cancers

Workup
- H&P
- Upper GI endoscopy and biopsy
- Chest/abdominal CT with oral and IV contrast
- Pelvic CT as clinically indicated
- PET/CT evaluation if no evidence of M1 disease
- CBC and chemistry profile
- Endoscopic ultrasound (EUS), if no evidence of M1 disease
- Endoscopic mucosal resection (EMR) may contribute to accurate staging of early stage cancers
- Nutritional assessment and counseling
- Biopsy of metastatic disease as clinically indicated
- HER-2-neu testing if metastatic adenocarcinoma is documented/suspected
- Bronchoscopy, if tumor is at or above the carina with no evidence of M1 disease
- Assign Siewert category
- Smoking cessation advice, counseling, and pharmacotherapy

Additional Evaluation
- Laparoscopy (optional) if no evidence of M1 disease, recommended only for patients with adenocarcinoma if the tumor is at the esophagogastric junction (EGJ)

Abbreviations: H&P, History and Physical Examination; HER, human epidermal growth factor receptor.

Adapted with permission from the NCCN Clinical Practice Guidelines in Oncology (NCCN Guidelines®) for Esophageal and Esophagogastric Junction Cancers V.2.2013. © 2013 National Comprehensive Cancer Network, Inc. All rights reserved. The NCCN Guidelines® and illustrations herein may not be reproduced in any form for any purpose without the express written permission of the NCCN. To view the most recent and complete version of the NCCN Guidelines, go online to NCCN.org. NATIONAL COMPREHENSIVE CANCER NETWORK®, NCCN®, NCCN GUIDELINES®, and all other NCCN Content are trademarks owned by the National Comprehensive Cancer Network, Inc.

which allows for selective deflation of the right lung during the thoracoscopic portion of the procedure. A nasogastric tube is placed while paying attention to the length of total tube inserted, as it is necessary to pull back the tube prior to creation of the gastric conduit. The patient is placed in the left lateral decubitus position. Appropriate preoperative antibiotics are administered; the patient is secured to the operating table. All pressure points are adequately padded, and the patient must have sequential compression garments applied to the lower extremities. Special consideration must be given by the surgeon for preoperative administration of methylprednisolone (10 mg/kg given 30 minutes prior to incision) to reduce postoperative pulmonary complications.[7] The shoulder of the right arm is externally rotated, and the arm is put at near full extension (near 160°). The table is tilted as far anteriorly as possible so that the patient is 45° from prone. The robot is positioned to the right and superior to the patient. The surgeon is located at the remote console.

Ports are placed in the intercostal spaces as follows (**Fig. 1**):

12 mm trocar in the fifth or sixth intercostal space in the posterior axillary line
8 mm robotic trocar in the third or the fourth intercostal space in the posterior axillary line immediately anterior to the scapula
8 mm robotic trocar in the seventh or eighth intercostal space in the posterior axillary line
Accessory: 12 mm sixth or seventh intercostal space in the anterior axillary line
Accessory: 5 mm third intercostal space in the anterior axillary line

Carbon dioxide at a pressure of 5 to 15 mm Hg is used to insufflate the thoracic cavity; this improves visibility by reducing cautery and harmonic smoke in the thoracic cavity and helps displace the lung away from the operative field. A 0° videoscope is placed through the 12 mm port in the fifth or 6th intercostal space in the posterior axillary line. The 12 mm accessory port is used for graspers, lung and diaphragm retractors, suctioning, and sutures for ligation of the thoracic duct. The 5 mm accessory trocar in the third intercostal space in the anterior axillary line is used for graspers and can also be used for suctioning.

INTRATHORACIC ESOPHAGEAL MOBILIZATION

The posterior perihilar aspect of the right lung is retracted anteriorly, exposing the esophagus. The esophagus is mobilized from the diaphragm to the thoracic inlet. Hook cautery and fenestrated blunt graspers are used to dissect along the anterior aspect of the esophagus from the pericardial bulge to the inferior pulmonary vein. The left pleura, hiatus, and pericardium are completely cleaned. All periesophageal nodes are taken en bloc, often requiring mobilization of the inferior pulmonary ligament and adherent lung, skeletonizing the pericardium, left pleura, both hila, and the hiatus. The azygos vein, if uninvolved, should be preserved. The thoracic duct is triply ligated with a permanent braided suture and taken en bloc as necessary with the esophagus.

The dissection continues into the neck by resecting the supra-azygos esophagus and periesophageal tissue. Electrocautery is used to score the pleura; ultrasonic shears are used to take the peritracheal nodes and divide the right vagus nerve. The ultrasonic shears are utilized to reduce the risk of injury to the recurrent laryngeal nerve by reducing the dispersion of energy into the surrounding tissues. The periesophageal tissues are resected from the peritracheal and cervical and continued into the thoracic inlet. The authors perform a series of multilevel intercostal bupivacaine blocks to anesthetize the area, 0.125% with epinephrine, from T2 to T10, and further injections around each of the port sites. Two to 3 drains are left after completion of the dissection: a 19F round fluted silastic drain is placed superior to the diaphragm and brought out through the lower accessory port incision, and a 28F chest tube and/or a second 19F round fluted silastic drain is placed in the superior aspect of the thoracic cavity and brought through the superior accessory port incision. The robot is disengaged from the patient and the remaining thoracic incisions are closed and dressed sterilely.

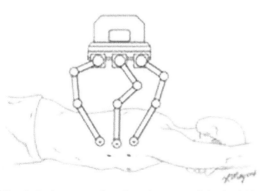

Fig. 1. Patients are placed semiprone and the bedside cart is brought in from the patient's left. The arm is positioned above the head and close to the patient's head. Two accessory ports are placed anteriorly, the more caudad port is 12 mm and the cephalad port is a 5 mm. (*Courtesy of* Nicholas Mayeux, Dallas, TX.)

Abdominal and Neck Phases

The second portion of the operation is performed after the patient is repositioned supine. Anesthesia reintubates the patient with a single-lumen endotracheal tube. Once the airway is secured, the patient's head is turned to the right, and the neck is extended. The neck and abdomen are prepared and draped in the standard fashion. A 5 to 8 cm transverse incision is made in the left neck 3 cm superior to the clavicle or alternatively along the lower anterior border of the sternocleidomastoid muscle. The dissection proceeds toward the cervical spine. The omohyoid is routinely divided to aid exposure. The esophagus has already been mobilized from the prior dissection and now has a Penrose drain passed around it for traction. The Penrose drain is secured, and the incision is packed with a moist laparotomy pad. Packing the neck wound helps prevent CO_2 leakage during abdominal insufflation.

A total of 6 abdominal ports are placed (**Fig. 2**):

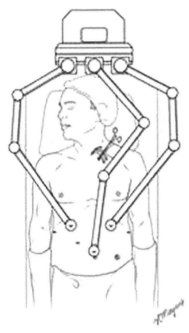

Fig. 2. Once the esophagus and periesophageal tissue has been fully mobilized from the diaphragm to the cervical esophagus, there is neck incision made just anterior to the sternocleidomastoid. After transecting the omohyoid, we dissect toward the anterior longitudinal spinous ligament. Since the dissection has already been performed there, it easily allows the passage of a Penrose drain around it; later used as a handle to pull the specimen up to the neck. Six laparoscopic ports are then placed. In the left lower quadrant ,we place a jejunostomy feeding tube. The bedside cart is brought in from the patient's head to create the gastric tube. (*Courtesy of* Nicholas Mayeux, Dallas, TX.)

Two 5 mm ports beneath each costal margin in the anterior axillary line

12 mm port at the right midclavicular line 2 to 3 cm above the umbilicus level

Two robotic 8 mm ports are placed 8 cm subcostally in the right and left midclavicular lines

12 mm viewing port is placed just cephalad to the umbilicus

The abdomen is insufflated with CO_2 to 15 mm Hg. A transcutaneous jejunal 10F feeding tube is placed 20 cm from the ligament of Treitz with T fasteners. The esophageal hiatus is exposed using a liver retractor through the right 5 mm accessory port. The robot is positioned at the head of the operating room table. The videoscope is placed through the 12 mm supraumbilical trocar, and the robot arms are placed through both of the 8 mm ports.

An ultrasonic cutting and coagulation generator is used to transect the lesser omentum and the short gastric arteries to the right gastroepiploic vein at the transverse mesentery. Great care is taken to preserve the right gastroepiploic arcade along its entirety. A Kocher maneuver is not necessary, but the pyloric attachments are transected to allow sufficient mobilization of the stomach. Lymph nodes are located at the splenic hilum, along the splenic artery to the origin of the left gastric artery, and along the common hepatic artery.

After the node dissection, the gastric conduit is constructed. First, to allow for clear first staple firing to prepare the gastric tube, the lesser curve of the gastric wall is cleared of all perigastric tissue 5 cm cephalad from the origin of the right gastric artery. A gastric tube with a diameter of 4 to 5 cm is created by firing approximately 10 loads of a thick linear tissue endostapler (staple height 4.1 mm or greater). A pyloroplasty is not required unless the patient has some obstruction; the authors usually inject 1 ml of botulinum toxin into each quadrant of the pylorus. The cephalad portion of the gastric tube is sutured to the distal end of the esophageal specimen with 2 sutures in a figure of 8 fashion. The chest tube suction and ventilation are temporarily held. The Penrose drain in the neck is used to pull the specimen carefully up through the neck incision until the gastric conduit reaches the neck. Great care is taken to avoid twisting of the gastric conduit. The anterior gastric conduit serosa is sutured to the crus of the diaphragm bilaterally using permanent braided suture in a figure of 8 fashion. The robot is moved away from the patient. The abdominal trocar sites are closed in the standard fashion.

The superior aspect of the esophagus is transected in the neck. An esophagogastrostomy is performed as a triangular side-to-side functional end-to-end stapled anastomosis. Before completion of the anastomosis, a nasogastric tube is manually directed distal to the anastomosis. A 75 × 4.1 mm linear endostapler and a 60 × 4.1 mm transverse stapler are used to create the anastomosis. A 10F flat drain is placed in the neck below the platysma but not directly touching the anastomosis. The neck is closed in layers with interrupted absorbable sutures (**Fig. 3**).

IMMEDIATE POSTOPERATIVE CARE

Patients undergoing robotic esophagectomy do not require routine admission to the surgical ICU. Patients may be safely managed on the floor unless their comorbidities mandate intensive care observation. Pain control is routinely achieved without narcotics by postoperative day 2. The nasogastric tube is left in place for 3 to 6 days. On postoperative day 6, an esophagram is performed. Patients with a normal esophagram are advanced to a diet consisting of 5 small meals a day. Patients with concern for an esophageal leak are kept on nothing by mouth, and an esophagram is repeated in 3 to 5 days. The chest tubes and the neck drain are removed after there is no longer a concern for a leak.

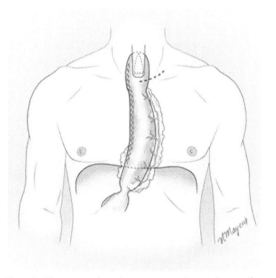

Fig. 3. The completed reconstruction allows for approximately a 300 ml stomach beneath the diaphragm. No pyloroplasty is performed. (*Courtesy of Nicholas Mayeux, Dallas, TX.*)

REHABILITATION AND RECOVERY

From meta-analysis by Clark and colleagues,[8] the reported 30-day mortality for robotic esophagectomy was 2.4% (3 of 126) with a hospital stay that ranged from 1 to 3 weeks (mean 15 days). Postoperative functional outcomes in terms of quality-of-life have yet to be reported in the literature.

CLINICAL RESULTS IN THE LITERATURE

The first reported 2-stage, 3-field robotic esophagolymphadenectomy for esophageal adenocarcinoma was published almost a decade ago.[9] This original technique has evolved with experience in an attempt to limit complications and further utilize the advantage of robotic dissection.[10] This technique allows for a complete lymphadenectomy under direct vision and for a cervical esophagogastric anastomosis. A neck anastomosis provides easier management of anastomotic leak and produces a more extensive proximal resection margin. For patients with locoregional esophageal carcinoma, radical surgical resection of the esophagus and any adjacent potentially involved tissues, as well as associated lymph nodes, provides the highest chance of achieving cure.[11] In contrast, the historical and open transhiatal esophagectomy carries less morbidity but is limited by the fact that the carinal and paratracheal nodes are not resected.[12] Currently, the sole commercially available computer-assisted surgical system (CAS) is the da Vinci Surgical System (Intuitive Surgical, Incorporated, Sunnyvale, CA). This system is able to provide a 3-dimensional view with up to an additional tenfold magnification of the operative field. When compared with traditional laparoscopy, the robot instruments are able to achieve 7 degrees of motion.[13] Additionally, it improves dexterity compared with the rigidity of standard thoracoscopic instruments. The computer system is able to filter the surgeon's natural tremor and scale motions to a predetermined degree, allowing for very precise movement. The camera is controlled by the surgeon, eliminating both the need for an assistant to hold the camera and unintentional movement of the visual field by the assistant. The disadvantages of the currently available robotic assisted procedures have been discussed in the literature.[13,14] The robot controls lack tactile feedback, and the bedside console is very large; additionally, the initial and maintenance costs of the robot are cumbersome, and the time required to properly dock the robot adds additional time to the procedure. The robot also physically separates the surgeon from patient, which is radical when compared with the traditional notion of surgery. However, this separation raises the possibility of a surgeon being able to operate remotely from any location in the world. Robotic surgery requires all members of the surgical team to learn new skills. No randomized controlled trials have been performed comparing robotic versus conventional surgical approaches for esophageal cancers. A recent systematic review of the literature by Clark and colleagues[8] failed to demonstrate an improvement in oncological outcomes with use of the robot. However, this review showed improvement in estimated blood loss, length of intensive care unit (ICU) stay, and total number of lymph nodes harvested when compared with open and laparoscopic techniques. The pulmonary complication rate and perioperative mortality were higher than the laparoscopic approach but similar to the open approach. A more extensive lymphadenectomy is important, as it has been associated with better survival.[15–18]

When comparing robot-assisted minimally invasive esophagectomy to thoracoscopic minimally invasive esophagectomy, a recent small retrospective review[19] demonstrated that there were no significant differences between operative time, blood loss, number of resected lymph nodes, postoperative complications, days of mechanical ventilation, length of ICU, or length of hospital stay. Weksler and colleagues concluded that the 2 approaches are equivalent in safety and efficacy. However, a prior systematic review by Clark and colleagues[8] of all published literature prior to April 2010 revealed that the mean number of specimen lymph nodes examined was from 12 to 38; the R0 (negative tumor margin rate) was from 76% to 100%, with 3 of the 5 series reporting R0 greater than or equal to 95%, and in the 2 series reporting disease recurrence beyond 6 months, the rate of recurrence was 17% and 38%, respectively. There were 7 case series that reported using the transthoracic approach. The conversion rate was 0% to 14%; 3 of the series reported no conversions. Two of the series reported major complication rates of approximately 30%, and another trial reported an overall rate of complications of 64%. The 30-day mortality was 0% in 5 of the 8 case series, with the others reporting a single death in each of the remaining series. Verhage and colleagues[20] compared the operative outcomes of the open, laparoscopic, and robotic approaches and found that there was no significant differences that could be discerned given the relatively small numbers and the operative time of approximately 6.2 hours. The estimated blood loss was similar for robotic and laparoscopic at 200 to 300 mL, but the open procedure appeared to be greater at nearly 600 mL. The reported ICU stay for the minimally invasive approaches was 4 to 6 days and possibly greater for the open approach at 8 days. The length of hospital stay was 21 days for the open approach, but the minimally invasive approach was 16 days, with no difference between the laparoscopic and robotic approaches. There were no apparent differences in the complication or mortality rates between the 3 approaches, being approximately 60% and 1% to 4%, respectively.

SUMMARY

The robotic modified-McKeown esophagectomy offers the potential of a thorough resection of mediastinal and upper esophageal disease. Most of the publications reporting robotic esophagectomy discuss the chest-only approach or the procedure as a part of the Ivor Lewis esophagectomy, so it is difficult to discern the role and outcomes of the McKeown approach. It appears that the anastomotic leak rate is greater with the McKeown, compared with the Ivor Lewis technique. Given the early experience and the currently available equipment, there does not appear to be any obvious superiority of the robotic esophagectomy to the laparoscopic/thoracoscopic approach. As the experience and equipment evolve, we should expect that the outcomes will continue to improve.

REFERENCES

1. Pohl H, Sirovich B, Welch HG. Esophageal adenocarcinoma incidence: are we reaching the peak? Cancer Epidemiol Biomarkers Prev 2010;19:1468.
2. Stahl M, Stuschke M, Lehmann N, et al. Chemoradiation with and without surgery in patients with locally advanced squamous cell carcinoma of the esophagus. J Clin Oncol 2005;23:2310.
3. Bedenne L, Michel P, Bouché O, et al. Chemoradiation followed by surgery compared with chemoradiation alone in squamous cancer of the esophagus: FFCD 9102. J Clin Oncol 2007;25:1160.
4. Biere SS, van Berge Henegouwen MI, Maas KW, et al. Minimally invasive versus open oesophagectomy for patients with oesophageal cancer: a multicentre, open-label, randomised controlled trial. Lancet 2012;379:1887.
5. Santillan AA, Farma JM, Meredith KL, et al. Minimally invasive surgery for esophageal cancer. J Natl Compr Canc Netw 2008;6:879.
6. Inoue J, Ono R, Makiura D, et al. Prevention of postoperative pulmonary complications through intensive preoperative respiratory rehabilitation in patients with esophageal cancer. Dis Esophagus 2013;26:68.

7. Sato N, Koeda K, Ikeda K, et al. Randomized study of the benefits of preoperative corticosteroid administration on the postoperative morbidity and cytokine response in patients undergoing surgery for esophageal cancer. Ann Surg 2002;236: 184–90.

8. Clark J, Sodergren M, Purkayastha S, et al. The role of robotic laparoscopy for oesophagogastric oncological resection; an appraisal of the literature. Dis Esophagus 2011;24:240–50.

9. Kernstine KH, DeArmond DT, Karimi M, et al. The robotic, 2-stage, 3-fieldesophagolymphadenectomy. J Thorac Cardiovasc Surg 2004;127:1847–9.

10. Kernstine KH, DeArmond DT, Karimi M, et al. The first series of completely robotic esophagectomies with three-field lymphadenectomy: initial experience. Surg Endosc 2007;21:2285–92.

11. Mariette C, Piessen G, Triboulet JP. Therapeutic strategies in oesophageal carcinoma: role of surgery and other modalities. Lancet Oncol 2007;8: 545–53.

12. Hulscher JB, van Sandick JW, de Boer AG, et al. Extended transthoracic resection compared with limited transhiatal resection for adenocarcinoma of the esophagus. N Engl J Med 2002;347:1662–9.

13. Watson TJ. Robotic esophagectomy: is it an advance and what is the future? Ann Thorac Surg 2008;85:S757–9.

14. Kastenmeier A, Gonzales HH, Gould JC. Robotic applications in the treatment of diseases of the esophagus. Surg Laparosc Endosc Percutan Tech 2012;22(4):304–9.

15. Greenstein AJ, Litle VR, Swanson SJ, et al. Effect of the number of lymph nodes sampled on postoperative survival of lymph-node negative esophageal cancer. Cancer 2008;112:1239.

16. Schwartz RE, Smith DD. Clinical impact of lymphadenectomy extent in resectable esophageal cancer. J Gastrointest Surg 2007;11:1384.

17. Peyre CG, Hagen JA, DeMeester SR, et al. The number of lymph nodes removed predicts survival in esophageal cancer: an international study on the impact of extent of surgical resection. Ann Surg 2008;248:549.

18. Risk NP, Ishwaran H, Rice TW, et al. Optimum lymphadenectomy for esophageal cancer. Ann Surg 2010;251:46.

19. Weksler B, Sharma P, Moudgill N, et al. Robot-assisted minimally invasive esophagectomy is equivalent to thoracoscopic minimally invasive esophagectomy. Dis Esophagus 2012;25:403–9.

20. Verhage RJ, Hazebroek EJ, Boone J, et al. Minimally invasive surgery compared to open procedures in esophagectomy for cancer: a systematic review of the literature. Minerva Chir 2009;64: 135–46.

Robotic-Assisted Minimally Invasive Esophagectomy
The Ivor Lewis Approach

Inderpal S. Sarkaria, MD*, Nabil P. Rizk, MD

KEYWORDS

- Esophageal cancer • Minimally invasive esophagectomy • Robotic surgery • Esophagectomy

KEY POINTS

- Robotic-assisted minimally invasive esophagectomy (RAMIE) is emerging as an alternative to minimally invasive esophagectomy (MIE).
- Early retrospective reports suggest RAMIE Ivor Lewis is feasible, with short-term outcomes equivalent to those of open surgery or standard MIE.
- Potential pitfalls and complications, in particular during airway dissection and anastomotic creation, are avoidable and should be recognized.
- Prospective trials investigating safety, outcomes, and quality-of-life profiles for RAMIE are currently accruing.

Videos of Hiatal dissection, Retrogastric dissection, Pyloroplasty, Conduit formation, Esophageal mobilization, Subcarinal dissection, Creation of anastomosis: securing stapler anvil, Creation of anastomosis: stapling and completion accompany this article at http://www.thoracic.theclinics.com/

INTRODUCTION: NATURE OF THE PROBLEM

In patients with benign or malignant disease requiring esophagectomy, minimally invasive approaches to resection have become increasingly used, with a growing body of data documenting excellent outcomes in these patients.[1–3] At least 1 randomized prospective study has cited decreased pulmonary complications and improved perioperative outcomes with minimally invasive esophagectomy (MIE) in comparison with open resection.[4]

Although robotic approaches to these operations have been described, the published experience with robotic-assisted minimally invasive esophagectomy (RAMIE) remains small. Studies cite a wide range of surgical approaches, with an equally variable quality in the reporting of technique and outcomes, including complications.

At the authors' institution a RAMIE approach was initiated in 2010 with the primary goals as follows: (1) to maximize patient safety; (2) to allow controlled introduction of robotic technology to already established procedures, with critical, prospective examination of outcomes and adverse events; and (3) if feasible, to develop a standardized procedure potentially portable to other centers and surgeons performing these operations.[5] The procedure resulting from this process is described herein.

Disclosures: The authors have no disclosures.
Thoracic Service, Department of Surgery, Memorial Sloan-Kettering Cancer Center, Weill Cornell Medical College, 1275 York Avenue, New York, NY 10065, USA
* Corresponding author.
E-mail address: sarkarii@mskcc.org

Thorac Surg Clin 24 (2014) 211–222
http://dx.doi.org/10.1016/j.thorsurg.2014.02.010
1547-4127/14/$ – see front matter © 2014 Elsevier Inc. All rights reserved.

SURGICAL TECHNIQUE
Preoperative Planning

All patients presenting with an endoscopy-confirmed and biopsy-confirmed diagnosis of esophageal carcinoma undergo rigorous preoperative evaluation to assess comorbidities and fitness for surgery. Staging is performed by means of computed tomography scanning of the chest, abdomen, and pelvis; endoscopic ultrasonography; and fluorodeoxyglucose-18 positron emission tomography scanning. Patients with early-stage lesions confined to the mucosa (T1a or less) are referred for diagnostic endoscopic mucosal resection and potentially therapeutic endoscopic resection with or without ablation of remaining Barrett mucosa. Patients with clinically early-stage lesions (T1b or T2 with no evidence of local lymph node metastases) are referred for surgery. Patients with clinically advanced local-regional disease (T3 and/or any N) are referred for induction chemotherapy and radiation, followed by surgical resection approximately 4 to 6 weeks after completion of treatment.

Preparation and Patient Positioning

The basic room setup for the abdominal and thoracic phases of the operation is depicted in **Fig. 1**. The robotic instrumentation cart is set up on the patient's right side, and the tower is set up on the left. The authors use a 4-arm robotic platform with 2 operating consoles. The operating surgeon and surgical trainee are positioned at the robotic consoles, and an assisting surgeon remains at the bedside. All patients receive an epidural catheter. An arterial line is placed routinely, and single-lung isolation with double-lumen tube intubation is performed routinely during the thoracoscopic phase. Upper endoscopy is performed before positioning, to assess the position of the tumor and the extent of gastric cardia and fundus involvement, if any.

For the abdominal phase, patients are placed supine on the operating table. The arms are placed at 45° on arm rests, and the patient is shifted to the right side of the bed to allow appropriate use of the liver retractor. Alternatively, to minimize interaction with the robotic assistant arm, the left arm may be tucked. A footboard is placed, and the patient is carefully secured to the table. Before the patient is prepped, the bed is briefly tested in steep reverse Trendelenburg position to confirm the stability of the patient on the table.

For the thoracic phase, the patient is placed in flexion in standard left lateral decubitus position, with the right side up and the upper arm in a neutral position. No prone positioning is used.

Surgical Approach and Port Placement

A combined sequential laparoscopic and thoracoscopic approach is used, as previously described.[5] For the abdominal approach, the operating table is turned 90° and brought into position to allow easy entry of the robotic cart and arms (da Vinci Surgical Robot; Intuitive Surgical Inc, Sunnyvale, CA) directly over the midline of the patient. A point approximately 1 to 2 cm above the xiphoid is marked in the midline. This point is used as a reference marker for the hiatus, the most cephalad of the abdominal phase, which all instrumentation

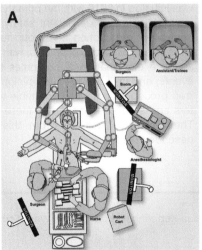 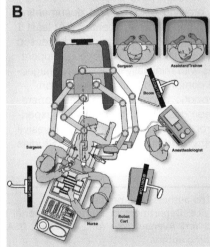

Fig. 1. Robotic-assisted minimally invasive esophagectomy (RAMIE) operating room setup for the abdominal (*A*) and thoracic (*B*) phases. (*Courtesy of* Memorial Sloan-Kettering Cancer Center, New York, NY; with permission.)

must be able to reach. A midline camera incision is marked preferably just above the umbilicus but no more than 23 cm from the supraxiphoid reference point. A left lateral subcostal 5-mm incision is marked for use by the robotic atraumatic grasper. A midclavicular 8-mm incision no more than 13 to 15 cm from the supraxiphoid reference point is marked in the left midabdomen. This port is for use with the ultrasonic shears (Harmonic Scalpel; Ethicon Inc, Somerville, NJ), which have a shorter operative length than most other instruments used with the current robotic system. An additional right lateral 5-mm subcostal port for placement of the liver retractor is marked, as well as an additional 8-mm midclavicular right midabdominal port for use with the bipolar atraumatic grasper. A 12-mm port is placed between the umbilical and the right midclavicular ports, and is used by the assistant for both suctioning and additional retraction. During later phases of the operation this port may be expanded to 15 mm, to allow entry of larger stapler sizes during gastric conduit formation, if needed. This port may also be used as an alternative camera entry site to improve visualization along the greater curve of the stomach during mobilization of the omentum and gastroepiploic arcade. Port placement is outlined in **Fig. 2**. To minimize arm collisions, it is important to maintain a distance of at least 9 to 10 cm between robotic ports.

The patient is prepped and draped, and the 12-mm camera port is placed in the midline using the direct Hassan trocar cutdown technique, with direct visualization of trocar entry into the peritoneal space. Peritoneal distension is then accomplished with pressurized CO_2 insufflation to 15 mm Hg at high flow rates. A standard 10-mm 30° laparoscope is used for the initial inspection of the peritoneal cavity and for identification of any metastatic disease, as well as for port placement. The left subcostal 5-mm port is placed next, under direct vision, as laterally as possible, followed by placement of the left 8-mm port. It is important to remeasure distances from the supraxiphoid reference point, as insufflation of the abdomen can result in differences from the initial measurement of 2 to 6 cm, depending on the abdominal girth of the patient. The right lateral 5-mm port is created for introduction of the liver retractor, which is placed under direct vision and secured with a static retraction device (MediFlex retractor; MediFlex, Islandia, NY). Finally, the right midclavicular 8-mm robotic port and 12-mm assistant port are placed. The center column of the robotic cart is brought over the midline of the patient, the patient is placed in optimum reverse Trendelenburg position (as allowable by the robotic cart), the robotic arms are docked to the ports, and the robotic instruments are placed into the peritoneal cavity under direct vision. It is important that once the ports are docked to the robotic arms, further positioning of the patient cannot occur without first undocking the arms.

For the thoracic phase, an insufflation needle with a saline-filled open syringe is placed into the chest, with water entry confirming safe intrapleural position. CO_2 insufflation is instituted at a pressure of 8 mm Hg. A standard laparoscopic 10-mm

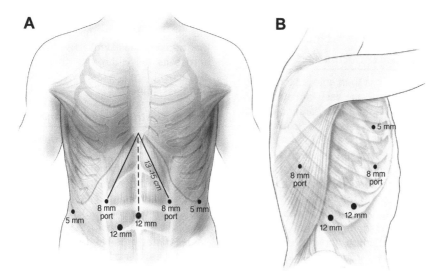

Fig. 2. RAMIE port placement for the abdominal (*A*) and thoracic (*B*) phases. (*Courtesy of* Memorial Sloan-Kettering Cancer Center, New York, NY; with permission.)

camera is placed into the obturator of the camera port, which is introduced into the chest in the eighth intercostal space in the mid to posterior axillary line under direct video guidance. The remaining ports are placed under direct intrathoracic visualization. A 5-mm robotic port is placed in the third intercostal space in the mid to posterior axillary line, and an 8-mm robotic port is placed in the fifth intercostal space. An additional 8-mm port is placed laterally in approximately the eighth or ninth interspace. A 12-mm assistant port is placed under direct vision at the diaphragmatic insertion. To avoid collisions with the bedside assistant, this port should lie midway between the camera port and the lateral 8-mm robotic port. The robot is docked to the ports, and the robotic camera is placed within the chest at a 30° downward orientation.

SURGICAL PROCEDURE: ABDOMINAL PHASE
Step 1: Initial Hiatal Dissection

Initial dissection is begun by opening the lesser sac and dissecting free the esophageal hiatus (Video 1). If a replaced left hepatic artery is encountered, it is clipped temporarily; the left liver lobe is assessed after a period of time and is often sacrificed if no vascular compromise to the liver is identified. For lower esophageal tumors, portions of the right or left crus may be dissected free and removed with the esophagus if cause for suspicion of tumor involvement is identified. Excessive mediastinal dissection should be minimized at this time to avoid entry into the pleural spaces, which may cause hemodynamic compromise and loss of intraperitoneal CO_2 insufflation. If this occurs, the surgeon should consider a low threshold for the performance of tube thoracostomy.

Step 2: Retrogastric Dissection

The retrogastric space is then entered through the lesser curve, and the robotic assistant arm is used to gently retract the stomach anteriorly, thus exposing the left gastric vascular pedicle (Video 2). Additional retraction by the bedside assistant is useful to completely expose this area. Dissection is begun along the superior border of the pancreas and splenic artery, posteriorly to the retroperitoneal planes, superiorly to the hiatus, and medially to the right partway along the common hepatic artery and then superiorly toward the hiatus. Thus, all retrogastric lymph nodes are dissected free circumferentially around the left gastric vascular pedicle. The celiac axis is carefully assessed for bulky adenopathy with persistent disease, the presence of which may preclude

resection. The authors prefer to partly skeletonize the proximal vascular pedicle, thus lifting all nodal-bearing tissue along with the specimen. The vascular pedicle is divided with an endovascular stapler introduced through the assistant port. Gentle retraction of the stomach by the robotic assistant arm allows for exposure and additional dissection of the left crus from the lesser gastric curve.

Step 3: Gastric Mobilization

Attention is next turned to the greater curve of the stomach, and the termination of the gastroepiploic arcade is identified (Video 3). The short gastric arteries are divided using the ultrasonic shears, with careful dissection of the gastrosplenic attachments and completion of the left crural mobilization. The lesser sac is then again entered through the greater omentum, and the gastric mobilization is completed to the level of the pylorus, taking great care to visualize and preserve the gastroepiploic arcade at all times. To better visualize the gastroepiploic vasculature, the left lateral robotic assistant arm can be used to gently retract the greater curve of the stomach medially and superiorly. This action also aids in identifying retrogastric adhesions, which must be lysed to completely mobilize the stomach.

Step 4: Pyloroplasty

To better visualize the pylorus, the left lateral robotic assistant arm is used to gently grasp the antrum of the stomach and retract it laterally to the left (Video 4). Retraction stitches are placed laterally across the pyloric muscle; these also aid in hemostasis of the Mayo vein. Orientation of the pylorus is maintained by gentle traction on the stitches by both the right robotic arm and the bedside assistant. The pylorus is opened across its full width with the ultrasonic shears, and closed transversely with 2-0 Vicryl with robotic assistance.

Step 5: Gastric Conduit Formation

In preparation for gastric tubularization, the left lateral robotic assistant arm is used to retract the most mobile portion of the gastric fundus toward the left upper quadrant, with an additional robotic grasper (Cadiere forceps) providing gentle inferior traction on the antrum (Video 5). The nasogastric tube is withdrawn into the esophagus. An endovascular stapler is used to divide the lesser curve vasculature at a point approximating the incisura. The gastric tube is constructed with multiple fires of the Endo gastrointestinal stapler, introduced through the 12-mm assistant port, with careful attention paid to proper orientation of the evolving conduit at all times. A final stapler fire divides the conduit from the specimen. The conduit is then re-approximated to the specimen with heavy suture to allow for properly oriented entry through the hiatus into the chest during the thoracoscopic phase of the operation. A standard laparoscopic feeding jejunostomy is placed, and the abdominal phase is completed.

SURGICAL PROCEDURE: THORACIC PHASE
Step 6: En Bloc Esophageal Mobilization

Using the 5-mm atraumatic robotic grasper, the lower lobe of the lung is retracted superior-laterally, and the inferior ligament is divided to the level of the inferior pulmonary vein (Video 6). The initial en bloc dissection is begun along the pericardium adjacent to the inferior vena cava. A combination of gentle blunt and sharp dissection readily allows the surgeon to completely mobilize the esophageal hiatus down to the contralateral pleura. Dissection is continued superiorly by first opening the mediastinal pleura along the hilum, with the lung retracted anterior-medially. Great care is taken to identify the airway early in this dissection and to carefully dissect free the sub-carinal lymph nodes. To avoid causing thermal injury, the surgeon must be careful to maintain distance between the dissection plane and the airway when using the ultrasonic shears, and use of alternative energy sources for dissection, such as the robotic bipolar Maryland forceps, is highly recommended (Video 7). The bedside assistant's use of thoracoscopic suction to maintain a clear surgical field aids in this dissection, as does careful mainte-nance of hemostasis with the robotic bipolar cautery forceps. Dissection is continued en bloc up until the level of the azygos vein, which is divided with an endovascular stapler. Use of a Penrose drain around the esophagus may aid in retraction and exposure, but is often not necessary. The vagus nerve is also divided at this level to avoid traction injury to the recurrent laryngeal nerve. The dissection is continued superiorly along the esophagus 3 to 4 cm above the azygos vein. The posterior mediastinal pleura is divided, and the posterior dissection is completed along the aorta to the level of the hiatus, with careful identi-fication and division of aortoesophageal perfo-rating arteries. Surgical clips placed through the assistant port are used liberally to seal lymphatic perforators. The thoracic duct is not routinely removed with the specimen but is ligated at the esophageal hiatus.

The conduit is carefully brought into the chest in proper orientation, with the lesser curve staple line facing laterally. The specimen and conduit are separated, and the conduit is reattached to the dia-phragm to prevent retraction into the abdomen dur-ing the remainder of the dissection. The specimen is retracted laterally and superiorly with the atrau-matic robotic grasper, and the deep dissection along the contralateral pleura and left mainstem bronchus is completed. Thus, all nodal-bearing tis-sue along the pericardium, airway, contralateral pleura, and aorta are removed with the specimen en bloc.

The esophagus is divided above the azygos vein, and the nasogastric tube is withdrawn prox-imally into the remaining proximal esophagus un-der direct vision. The posterior 8-mm robotic port is extended to a mini access incision 4 cm in length, and a wound protector device is placed. The specimen is removed and evaluated by frozen section to assess margins.

Step 7: Creation of Circular Stapled Anastomosis

Securing the stapler anvil
The orifice of the open esophagus is gently re-tracted and held open with the aid of the atrau-matic robotic grasper by the bedside assistant (Video 8). The anvil of the end anastomotic stapler is grasped with a strong robotic forceps (Prograsp; Intuitive Surgical) and carefully introduced into the distal open esophagus. A robotically sewn "baseball-stitch" purse-string suture is placed to hold the anvil in place, as well as a second, more superficial robotically sewn purse-string suture as reinforcement.

Stapler insertion and firing
The conduit is released from the diaphragm and the conduit is brought gently into the chest (Video 9), which can usually be accomplished with the robotic instruments. If there is any diffi-culty in advancing the conduit, consideration should be given to performing this maneuver with standard laparoscopic instruments from the bedside to avoid unrecognized tension and injury to the gastric wall or vascular supply. A gastro-tomy is performed at the most proximal portion of the conduit, and carefully held open with the assistance of robotic retraction and the bedside assistant. The end-anastomotic stapler is intro-duced through the mini access incision and care-fully placed into the proximal conduit. The conduit is carefully advanced into the chest and positioned, and the stapler spike is brought out along the greater curve in close apposition to the gastroepiploic arcade. The spike and anvil are married, and the anastomosis is created. The nasogastric tube is advanced into the gastric

conduit under direct vision. The proximal redundant conduit and gastrotomy are closed with an Endo gastrointestinal stapler. Care is taken to allow a distance of at least 2 cm between the anastomotic and gastrotomy closure staple lines. The procedure is completed with the placement of a chest tube, as well as a Jackson-Pratt drain adjacent to the anastomosis posteriorly.

Immediate postoperative care

Patients are extubated in the operating room and remain overnight in a step-down unit. Early ambulation on the first postoperative day is routine. Tube feeding is begun and slowly advanced on postoperative day 2. Nasogastric tubes are left in place for 5 to 7 days. An esophagogram is performed on removal of the nasogastric tubes to assess for leak; a liquid diet is begun in the absence of leak or if an identified leak is small and contained. Patients are discharged on days 7 to 9 and return to the clinic in approximately 3 weeks, at which time the perianastomotic drain is removed; the feeding jejunostomy is removed if the patient is tolerating a soft diet.

CLINICAL RESULTS IN THE LITERATURE

Experience with RAMIE is in its infancy. Although growing, the literature pertaining to RAMIE remains sparse and is limited to case reports and early institutional case series. These reports are summarized in **Table 1**. The vast majority of series detail a modified McKeown (3-hole) or transhiatal approach[6–22] lymph node retrieval was 20 (range, 3–38).

Cerfolio and colleagues[23] reported the first series of cases with an intrathoracic anastomosis, which comprised 22 patients undergoing Ivor Lewis resection with robotic assistance in the chest and standard laparoscopy in the abdomen. Among the initial 6 patients undergoing a posterior stapled and anterior hand-sewn anastomosis, the investigators noted significant morbidity, with anastomotic leak, gastric conduit leak, and 5 reoperations during the hospital stay. Among the remaining 16 patients, who underwent robotically hand-sewn 2-layer anastomosis, there was a significant decrease in morbidity; Cerfolio and colleagues advocate this anastomosis for intrathoracic robotic approaches. In a subset of 17 of 21 patients undergoing RAMIE, the authors' group described the first total robotic Ivor Lewis RAMIE procedure with robotic assistance in both the chest and abdomen (the remaining 4 patients underwent total RAMIE with a 3-hole approach).[5] Median operative time was 556 minutes, which dropped to 414 minutes for the last 5 cases, and

median lymph node harvest was 20 (range, 10–49). Intrathoracic anastomoses were performed with standard circular anastomotic staplers, with the anvil secured with robotically placed purse-string sutures. Anastomotic leaks occurred in 3 patients. Of concern, 3 patients developed airway fistulas, 1 of which resulted in respiratory failure and death on postoperative day 70. The authors believe that this may have been caused by the use of rigid thermal devices, such as the ultrasonic shears, and fixed tangential instrument angles, combined with a lack of haptic feedback, causing unrecognized indirect abrasion to the airway. Although these complications have been largely unreported, personal communication regarding similar complications from experienced surgeons at other high-volume esophageal centers performing RAMIE have substantiated these concerns. The authors have since tailored their approach to use available wristed bipolar energy sources (Maryland Bipolar; Intuitive Surgical) during the subcarinal dissection. In an as yet unpublished follow-up experience with more than 80 RAMIE operations, the authors have encountered no further such complications, and operative outcomes have been excellent, with no additional mortality.

De la Fuente and colleagues[24] have also reported on a series of 50 RAMIE cases with intrathoracic anastomosis, approximately half of which underwent total robotic Ivor Lewis procedures. The remainder underwent RAMIE with thoracic robotic assistance and hybrid abdominal procedures with standard laparoscopy or hand assistance. Anastomoses were created with circular staplers using a transoral 25-mm anvil. Reported operative outcomes were excellent, with no mortality, 1 anastomotic leak, and a median lymph node retrieval of 19 (range, 8–63). In a report from the same institution that was aimed at defining the learning curve for their RAMIE procedure, Hernandez and colleagues[25] reported significant reductions in mean operative time, from 514 minutes to 397 minutes, after the completion of 20 cases. These findings are largely in accord with the authors' findings from Memorial Sloan-Kettering Cancer Center: in an initial cohort of 45 patients undergoing RAMIE, there was intertertile improvement between successive cohorts of 15 patients in rates of major complications, lymph node retrieval, conversions to open procedures, and operative time (from approximately 600 minutes to 370 minutes, with a median operative time for the last 5 patients of less than 300 minutes [Inderpal S. Sarkaria, MD, personal communication, 2014]). These data suggest a case requirement of approximately 30 cases to

Table 1
Summary of reports on robotic-assisted minimally invasive esophagectomy

Authors,[Ref.] Year	Surgical Approach	Hybrid vs Total Robotic	Robotic Approach	No.	Procedure Time (Range), min	EBL (Range), mL	LOS (Range), d	Lymph Nodes	Overall Morbidity, 30-day Mortality, %	Comment
Melvin et al,[6] 2002	Ivor Lewis	NR	NR	1	462	NR	12	NR	NR	NR
Horgan et al,[19] 2003	Transhiatal	Total	L	1	246	50	7	NR	NR	NR
Giulianotti et al,[7] 2003	3-Hole	Hybrid	T	5	490 (420–540)[a]	NR	NR	NR	NR, 20	Death from anastomotic leak
Kernstine et al,[10] 2004	3-Hole	Total	T and L	1	660	900	8	NR	0, 0	
Bodner et al,[8] 2004	3-Hole	Hybrid	T	4	173 (171–190)	NR	NR	NR	0, NR	
Espat et al,[20] 2005[b]	Transhiatal	Total	L	15	274 (180–360)[a]	53 (NR)[a]	NR	NR	NR, 0	
Ruurda et al,[11] 2005[c]	3-Hole	Hybrid	T	22	180 (120–240)[d]	400 (150–700)[d]	18 (11–182)	NR	64, 5	14% anastomotic leak, 5% gastrostomy leak, 14% VC paralysis, 50% pulmonary complications, death from TE fistula, 1 intraoperative complication noted but not described

(continued on next page)

Table 1
(continued)

Authors,[Ref.] Year	Surgical Approach	Hybrid vs Total Robotic	Robotic Approach	No.	Procedure Time (Range), min	EBL (Range), mL	LOS (Range), d	Lymph Nodes	Overall Morbidity, 30-day Mortality, %	Comment
van Hillegersberg et al,[12] 2006[c]	3-Hole	Hybrid	T	21	451 (370–550)	950 (250–5300)	18 (11–182)	20 (9–30)	NR, 5	48% pulmonary complications (14% acute lung injury), 14% anastomotic leak, death from TE fistula
Dapri et al,[9] 2006	3-Hole	Hybrid	T	2	NR	NR	7, 12	18, 21	0, 0	
Kernstine et al,[17] 2007	3-Hole	Hybrid / Total	T / T and L	6 / 8	NR / 672 (570–780)	NR / 275 (50–950)	22 (8–72)	18 (10–32)	29, 7	Intraoperative airway injury, bilateral VC paralysis, 7% anastomotic leak
Anderson et al,[18] 2007	3-Hole / Transhiatal / Ivor Lewis	Total / Total / Hybrid	T and L / L / L	22 / 1 / 2	480 (391–646)	350 (100–1600)	11 (5–64)	22 (10–49)	32, 0	4 (16%) anastomotic leak
Braumann,[27] 2008	NR	NR	NR	4	60 (55–240)	NR	29 (13–31)	NR	NR	
Galvani & Horgan,[21] 2005[b]	Transhiatal	Hybrid	L	18	267 (180–365)[a]	54 (10–150)	10 (4–38)	14 (7–27)[a]	50, 0	33% anastomotic leak, 33% anastomotic stricture

Boone et al,[13] 2009c	3-Hole	Hybrid	T	47	450 (360–550)	625 (150–5300)	18 (10–182)	29	NR, 6	21% anastomotic leak, 45% pulmonary complications, 49% stage IVa, TE fistula
Kim et al,[16] 2010	3-Hole	Hybrid	T	21	410 (NR)	150 (50–2300)	21 (11–45)	12 (NR)	52, 0	19% anastomotic leak, 29% VC paralysis, surgeon with no prior thoracoscopic experience
Puntambekar et al,[15] 2011	3-Hole	Hybrid	T	32	210 (180–300)a	80 (40–200)a	9 (5–20)	36 (NR)	NR, NR	9% anastomotic leak, 6% pulmonary complications
Weksler et al,[14] 2011	3-Hole	Hybrid	T	11	445 (306–536)	150 (50–600)	7 (5–16)	19 (10–47)	NR, 9	Death from anastomotic breakdown and respiratory failure
Dunn et al,[22] 2013	Transhiatal	Total	L	40	311	100 (25–300)	9 (6–36)	20 (3–38)	NR, 3	25% anastomotic leak, 68% anastomotic stricture, 35% VC paralysis (all temporary)

(continued on next page)

Table 1
(continued)

Authors,[Ref.] Year	Surgical Approach	Hybrid vs Total Robotic	Robotic Approach	No.	Procedure Time (Range), min	EBL (Range), mL	LOS (Range), d	Lymph Nodes	Overall Morbidity, 30-day Mortality, %	Comment
Cerfolio et al,[23] 2013	Ivor Lewis	Hybrid	T	22	367 (290–453)	75 (40–800)	7 (6–32)	18 (15–28)	23, 0	Hand-sewn intrathoracic anastomosis, 1 anastomotic leak, 1 gastric conduit leak, 5 reoperations during same hospital stay, conversion for staple line dehiscence
de la Fuente et al,[24] 2013	Ivor Lewis	Total	L and T	50	445 (NR)[a]	146 (NR)[a]	9 (6–35)	19 (8–63)	28, NR	1 anastomotic leak, 1 gastric conduit leak, no in-hospital mortality
Sarkaria et al,[5] 2013	Ivor Lewis 3-Hole	Total Total	L and T T and L	17 4	556 (395–626)	300	10 (7–70)	20 (10–49)	24, 5	14% anastomotic leak, 14% airway fistulas

Abbreviations: EBL, estimated blood loss; L, laparoscopy; LOS, length of stay; NR, not recorded; T, thoracoscopy; TE, tracheoesophageal; VC, vocal cord.
  [a] Reported as mean.
  [b] Overlapping patient cohorts.
  [c] Overlapping patient cohorts.
  [d] Thoracoscopic portion only.

overcome the greater part of the learning curve for the RAMIE procedure.

There are no large series of RAMIE, and no case-control series comparing RAMIE to standard MIE. However, the level of evidence remains preliminary, with only a single meta-analysis by Clark and colleagues,[26] which indicated a 30% complication rate, 2.4% operative mortality, and 18% anastomotic leak rate in 60 patients undergoing RAMIE by various approaches.

At present, no prospective data comparing RAMIE with standard laparoscopic or open procedures exist. At Memorial Sloan-Kettering Cancer Center, the authors are actively accruing a prospective quality-of-life and outcomes trial comparing RAMIE with open esophagectomy (ClinicalTrials.gov: NCT01558648). In addition, a prospective, randomized controlled trial comparing complications and outcomes in RAMIE versus open transthoracic esophagectomy (also known as the ROBOT trial) is under way in the Netherlands, with an expected completion date of 2015 (ClinicalTrials.gov: NCT01544790).

SUMMARY

RAMIE Ivor Lewis is a technically demanding, but feasible approach to esophageal resection. It requires stringent patient selection and a multidisciplinary effort. Additional outcome data and further studies to evaluate differences between RAMIE and standard MIE including, but not limited to perioperative outcomes, cost implications and long-term oncologic outcomes in esophageal cancer must be undertaken. Although care must be taken during the learning phase of these operations to avoid known pitfalls and complications, RAMIE appears to be an equivalent alternative to standard MIE and open esophageal resections.

SUPPLEMENTARY DATA

Videos related to this article can be found online at http://dx.doi.org/10.1016/j.thorsurg.2014.02.010.

REFERENCES

1. Lazzarino AI, Nagpal K, Bottle A, et al. Open versus minimally invasive esophagectomy: trends of utilization and associated outcomes in England. Ann Surg 2010;252(2):292–8.
2. Luketich J, Pennathur A, Catalano PJ, et al. Results of a phase II multicenter study of minimally invasive esophagectomy (Eastern Cooperative Oncology Group Study E2202). J Clin Oncol 2009;27(15S): 4516.
3. Luketich JD, Pennathur A, Awais O, et al. Outcomes after minimally invasive esophagectomy: review of over 1000 patients. Ann Surg 2012;256(1):95–103.
4. Biere SS, van Berge Henegouwen MI, Maas KW, et al. Minimally invasive versus open oesophagectomy for patients with oesophageal cancer: a multicentre, open-label, randomised controlled trial. Lancet 2012;379(9829):1887–92.
5. Sarkaria IS, Rizk NP, Finley DJ, et al. Combined thoracoscopic and laparoscopic robotic-assisted minimally invasive esophagectomy using a four-arm platform: experience, technique and cautions during early procedure development. Eur J Cardiothorac Surg 2013;43(5):e107–15.
6. Melvin WS, Needleman BJ, Krause KR, et al. Computer-enhanced robotic telesurgery. Initial experience in foregut surgery. Surg Endosc 2002;16(12): 1790–2.
7. Giulianotti PC, Coratti A, Angelini M, et al. Robotics in general surgery: personal experience in a large community hospital. Arch Surg 2003; 138(7):777–84.
8. Bodner J, Wykypiel H, Wetscher G, et al. First experiences with the da Vinci operating robot in thoracic surgery. Eur J Cardiothorac Surg 2004; 25(5):844–51.
9. Dapri G, Himpens J, Cadiere GB. Robot-assisted thoracoscopic esophagectomy with the patient in the prone position. J Laparoendosc Adv Surg Tech A 2006;16(3):278–85.
10. Kernstine KH, DeArmond DT, Karimi M, et al. The robotic, 2-stage, 3-field esophagolymphadenectomy. J Thorac Cardiovasc Surg 2004;127(6):1847–9.
11. Ruurda JP, Draaisma WA, van Hillegersberg R, et al. Robot-assisted endoscopic surgery: a four-year single-center experience. Dig Surg 2005; 22(5):313–20.
12. van Hillegersberg R, Boone J, Draaisma WA, et al. First experience with robot-assisted thoracoscopic esophagolymphadenectomy for esophageal cancer. Surg Endosc 2006;20(9):1435–9.
13. Boone J, Schipper ME, Moojen WA, et al. Robot-assisted thoracoscopic oesophagectomy for cancer. Br J Surg 2009;96(8):878–86.
14. Weksler B, Sharma P, Moudgill N, et al. Robot-assisted minimally invasive esophagectomy is equivalent to thoracoscopic minimally invasive esophagectomy. Dis Esophagus 2011;25:403–9.
15. Puntambekar SP, Rayate N, Joshi S, et al. Robotic transthoracic esophagectomy in the prone position: experience with 32 patients with esophageal cancer. J Thorac Cardiovasc Surg 2011;142(5):1283–4.
16. Kim DJ, Hyung WJ, Lee CY, et al. Thoracoscopic esophagectomy for esophageal cancer: feasibility and safety of robotic assistance in the prone position. J Thorac Cardiovasc Surg 2010;139(1): 53–9.e1.

17. Kernstine KH, DeArmond DT, Shamoun DM, et al. The first series of completely robotic esophagectomies with three-field lymphadenectomy: initial experience. Surg Endosc 2007;21(12):2285–92.

18. Anderson C, Hellan M, Kernstine K, et al. Robotic surgery for gastrointestinal malignancies. Int J Med Robot 2007;3(4):297–300.

19. Horgan S, Berger RA, Elli EF, et al. Robotic-assisted minimally invasive transhiatal esophagectomy. Am Surg 2003;69(7):624–6.

20. Espat NJ, Jacobsen G, Horgan S, et al. Minimally invasive treatment of esophageal cancer: laparoscopic staging to robotic esophagectomy. Cancer J 2005;11(1):10–7.

21. Galvani C, Horgan S. Robots in general surgery: present and future. Cir Esp 2005;78(3):138–47 [in Spanish].

22. Dunn DH, Johnson EM, Morphew JA, et al. Robot-assisted transhiatal esophagectomy: a 3-year single-center experience. Dis Esophagus 2013; 26(2):159–66.

23. Cerfolio RJ, Bryant AS, Hawn MT. Technical aspects and early results of robotic esophagectomy with chest anastomosis. J Thorac Cardiovasc Surg 2013;145(1):90–6.

24. de la Fuente SG, Weber J, Hoffe SE, et al. Initial experience from a large referral center with robotic-assisted Ivor Lewis esophagogastrectomy for oncologic purposes. Surg Endosc 2013;27(9): 3339–47.

25. Hernandez JM, Dimou F, Weber J, et al. Defining the Learning Curve for Robotic-assisted Esophagogastrectomy. J Gastrointest Surg 2013;17(8):1346–51.

26. Clark J, Sodergren MH, Purkayastha S, et al. The role of robotic assisted laparoscopy for oesophago-gastric oncological resection; an appraisal of the literature. Dis Esophagus 2011;24(4):240–50.

27. Braumann C, Jacobi CA, Menenakos C, et al. Robotic-assisted laparoscopic and thoracoscopic surgery with the da Vinci system: a 4-year experience in a single institution. Surg Laparosc Endosc Percutan Tech 2008;18(3):260–6.

Robotic Benign Esophageal Procedures

Jennifer M. Hanna, MD, MBA, Mark W. Onaitis, MD*

KEYWORDS

- Achalasia • Fundoplication • Paraesophageal hernia • Robotic surgery
- Benign esophageal disease

KEY POINTS

- Robotic master-slave devices can assist surgeons to perform minimally invasive esophageal operations with approaches that have already been demonstrated using laparoscopy and thoracoscopy.
- Robotic-assisted surgery for benign esophageal disease is described for the treatment of achalasia, epiphrenic diverticula, refractory reflux, paraesophageal hernias, duplication cysts, and benign esophageal masses, such as leiomyomas.
- Indications and contraindications for robotic surgery in benign esophageal disease should closely approximate the indications for laparoscopic and thoracoscopic procedures.
- Given the early application of the technology and paucity of clinical evidence, there are currently no procedures for which robotic esophageal surgery is the clinically proven preferred approach.

INTRODUCTION

As a pliable muscular tube that spans 3 body compartments in close proximity to the great vessels, the esophagus and its anatomic design impart formidable challenges to the surgeon. Operative approaches are made more difficult by the secondary physiologic insult inherent in prolonged operations that traverse both sides of the diaphragm.

Pulmonary complications historically provide impetus for evolving surgical approaches to the esophagus. Minimally invasive techniques limit mechanical and physiologic stress. Despite potentially increased technical difficulty, laparoscopy and video-assisted thoracoscopic surgery result in decreased hospital stay, rapid recovery, and decreased perioperative morbidity.

Robotic master-slave devices are relatively new tools in the surgeon's armamentarium. With port size equivalent to those of other minimally invasive techniques, the theoretical advantages of the da Vinci system are based on the application of improved 3-dimensional visualization with 10-fold magnification. The surgical arms allow fine dissection and suturing with movements similar to those of human wrists, augmented with scaling ability and tremor elimination.

This article describes robotic approaches to benign esophageal pathologic conditions. Several benign esophageal disorders are best treated with surgical intervention. Examined in detail are the most common of these that are amenable to minimally invasive surgery with robotic assistance.

HISTORY AND GENERAL CONSIDERATIONS
The Development of Robotic Esophageal Surgery

Minimally invasive surgical techniques have been applied to essentially all aspects of general and thoracic surgery since their introduction in the 1980s. Success with other minimally invasive

Disclosures: I am a proctor for Intuitive Surgical.
Division of Cardiovascular and Thoracic Surgery, Department of Surgery, Duke University Medical Center, Box 3305, Erwin Road, Durham, NC 21170, USA
* Corresponding author. Department of Surgery, Duke University Medical Center, Box 3304 Medical Center, Durham, NC 27710.
E-mail address: mark.onaitis@duke.edu

Thorac Surg Clin 24 (2014) 223–229
http://dx.doi.org/10.1016/j.thorsurg.2014.02.004
1547-4127/14/$ – see front matter © 2014 Elsevier Inc. All rights reserved.

approaches has facilitated the application of robotic devices to esophageal procedures. These robotic-assisted esophageal operations are still in the early stages of development, and typically mirror the approaches that have been clinically successful for thoracoscopy and laparoscopy.

A clear timeline describing the evolution of robotic technology in gastrointestinal surgery is complicated by the differences in the release of devices in the United States and Europe. Although Himpens and colleagues[1] performed the first telesurgical laparoscopic cholecystectomy in 1997, the Food and Drug Administration of the United States did not approve a telesurgical device for use in general surgery until July 2000. Reports of robotic-assisted esophageal surgery began to surface shortly after the device was released for general use, and generally paralleled the techniques for performing the laparoscopic or thoracoscopic procedures.

Advantages and Disadvantages of Robotic Esophageal Surgery

Clinically proven advantages of robotic surgery are limited but, as with laparoscopy and thoracoscopy, will most likely be elucidated in patients with limited physiologic reserve and challenging anatomy.

Robotic surgery is most advantageous in a narrow interior field where the benefits of the wristed movements of the endoinstruments are maximized. As the operative target is located at a greater intracorporeal distance from the instrument port site, tremors that would normally increase are filtered by the computer system, and movements are scaled accordingly.

These mechanical advantages have notable potential in esophageal surgery whereby meticulous dissection and identification of proper tissue planes are of utmost importance. These tissue planes are already challenging to manipulate because of the characteristics of the esophageal fatty submucosa and mucosa. Difficulties increase as the population presenting for surgery becomes older, with an increased prevalence of previous instrumentation.

The lack of haptic feedback is a particularly important consideration when evaluating a patient for possible adhesions and access to the esophagus. Thoracoscopic and laparoscopic manipulation generally affords the operator some degree of tactile feedback so that if unexpected resistance is encountered outside the visual field, it can be quickly and appropriately addressed with repositioning of both the instruments and the camera. Although visual cues can mitigate some of the limitations of the robotic device in the operative field, there are no corresponding safeguards for the path of the arms as they travel between the body wall and the robotic visual field.

Whereas laparoscopy and thoracoscopy are plagued by a fulcrum effect at the distal limits of instrumentation, the dexterity of the robotic wristed movements is maintained throughout the dissection. These dexterous advantages only exist for the endowrists and not the external robotic joints. A large joint exists at a fixed angle to the device shaft immediately outside the body; robotic instruments are plagued not only by the same fulcrum limitations as are traditional minimally invasive instruments but also by external collisions of the machinery. As the hiatus is fixed, and the esophagus is a linear organ, robotic esophageal surgery is feasible in that the target anatomy can be placed in a line between the robot cart and the camera, thus minimizing collisions between instruments.

Operating-Room Setup

All members of the nursing team must be familiar with all aspects of the system, including video setup, movement of the robot itself, management of the console, and instrument draping. Indeed, robotic esophageal surgery is a careful, premeditated procedure that not only entails a preoperative workup but also institutional guidelines and staff training on every level.

The robotic cart weighs 550 kg and takes up a considerable amount of space in the operating theater. Room selection is important. The device must have a clear path to the required operative field, and the arms must be able to function without intracorporeal or extracorporeal restrictions. Unlike laparoscopy, whereby the angle of the operator can be easily changed, the robotic system is at a fixed angle in reference to the patient.

Diagnosis and Assessment

Each series of radiologic and endoscopic tests must be tailored for the patient and disease entity. Preoperative evaluations are based on clinical history and examination. The esophageal wall is not normally seen on plain films unless the lumen is distended with air. Demonstration of the azygoesophageal line and esophagopleural stripe may indicate wall thickening from conditions such as diffuse esophageal spasm or infiltration by tumor. Although chest radiography may help define pulmonary status, an evaluation before minimally invasive surgery requires adjunctive radiographic studies.

A barium swallow continues to maintain an essential role in the workup of patients with esophageal disease. This study allows excellent demonstration of both anatomy and motor function. Esophageal manometry and 24-hour esophageal pH monitoring are also needed to further evaluate peristalsis and pressures in the lower esophageal sphincter. In general, no additional diagnostic procedures are necessary for robotic esophageal surgery in comparison with laparoscopic and open approaches.

Specific Robotic Surgical Procedures

All procedures are performed under general anesthesia. Double-lumen endotracheal tubes for selective ventilation are necessary for transthoracic procedures. Additional blood-pressure monitoring with an arterial line is used for patients with selective lung ventilation or those with a significant cardiac history. An orogastric tube and esophageal temperature probe are initially placed. Foley catheters are used for procedures that are anticipated to last longer than 2 hours.

Similarly to thoracoscopic approaches, robotic esophageal procedures are facilitated with pulmonary insufflation and ipsilateral lung collapse. Insufflation increases esophageal exposure by distending the mediastinum, compressing the ipsilateral lung, and removing cautery smoke. Cautery is set on coagulate at a device level between 5 and 20 depending on proximity to neurovascular structures. Insufflation pressures are typically set at 15 mm Hg for abdominal procedures and 7 mm Hg for thoracic procedures.

ABDOMINAL PROCEDURES
Robotic-Assisted Laparoscopic Port Placement

In operations during which access to the hiatus is desired, the authors use the incision set depicted in **Fig. 1**. As **Fig. 1** illustrates, Hasson access is achieved superior to the umbilicus. Insufflation is performed here, and 8-mm robot ports are placed in right and left subcostal locations. Between the Hasson port and the right robotic arm, a 12-mm Step port is placed for assistant access. In a low right subcostal location, a 5-mm Step port is placed. Through this port a Nathanson retractor is placed to retract the left lateral section of the liver. A Fastclamp device is used to anchor this retractor.

Achalasia

With reported success rates of approximately 90%, many large institutions now favor minimally invasive surgical myotomy over the open

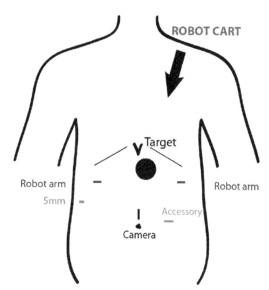

Fig. 1. Robotic-assisted laparoscopic port placement.

technique for long-term treatment of achalasia.[2,3] Thoracoscopic and laparoscopic approaches are technically advanced procedures, each with inherent difficulties. Although the submucosal plane is often easy to detect, the distal extent of the myotomy can be difficult to ascertain during a thoracoscopic approach because dissection of the tissue surrounding the gastroesophageal junction is at the limit of visualization and instrumentation. The strictures and fibrosis of the distal esophagus that sometimes ensue with balloon dilatation complicate surgical dissection. In the authors' opinion, the robotic approach from the abdomen maximizes visualization and precision.

As stated earlier, the workup for a patient with achalasia does not differ from that performed when laparoscopic or open surgery is performed. At the commencement of the case, esophagogastroduodenoscopy is performed to assess the extent of disease and to rule out other abnormality. Once the ports depicted in **Fig. 1** are inserted, the patient is placed in steep reverse Trendelenburg, and a 30-down robotic camera is placed. Using a fenestrated bipolar instrument in the left robotic arm and a spatula or hook cautery in the right robotic arm, the right crus is mobilized. The esophagus is dissected, taking care not to injure either phrenic nerve. The anterior phrenic nerve is elevated with the gastroesophageal fat pad. Dissection is carried anteriorly into the chest. The excellent robotic vision and wristed instruments make division of the longitudinal and circular muscle fibers straightforward. The mucosa is spared. In general, the myotomy is performed up to the inferior pulmonary veins and 2 cm onto the stomach. Esophagoscopy is again performed at the conclusion of the myotomy to assess for any undivided fibers. The authors generally perform an anterior Dor fundoplication using 2-0 Ticron sutures, a large suture-cut needle driver in the right robotic arm, and a large suture driver in the left robotic arm. The robotic vessel sealer or Harmonic scalpel may be used to take down a few short gastric vessels to facilitate the fundoplication.

Although large series do not exist, robotic esophageal myotomy is typically performed in 2 to 3 hours with excellent results and few complications.[4,5] In their description of a larger robotic experience, Giulianotti and colleagues[4] reported the use of the da Vinci robot to perform 5 esophageal myotomies with Dor fundoplication for achalasia. Melvin and colleagues[5] reported the use of the robot for 9 Heller myotomies. The authors' experience is similar to that of these investigators. Although the myotomy is subjectively easier using the robot, cost-effectiveness regarding laparoscopic Heller is yet to be addressed.

Epiphrenic Diverticulum

Diverticula can occur along the length of the esophagus and are classified according to location, pathogenesis, and morphology. Granulomatous mediastinal paraesophageal nodal disease results in traction diverticula, usually in the middle third of the esophagus. These true diverticula are of surgical importance only when ongoing mediastinal inflammation results in a fistulous communication with intrathoracic structures.

Thoracic pulsion diverticula typically occur with an associated motor disorder, and can be treated with a variety of transthoracic approaches. Resection and myotomy of asymptomatic epiphrenic diverticula are controversial. Heller introduced the open myotomy in 1913. Zaaijer[6] added a fundoplication in 1923. Although variations on the extent of the myotomy and the type of wrap evolved, the surgical approaches remained relatively unchanged until laparoscopic and thoracoscopic myotomies were reported by the groups of Shimi[7] and Pelligrini,[8] respectively.

Resection and myotomy for epiphrenic diverticulum are challenging procedures in either the chest or the abdomen. The authors have used a robot-assisted laparoscopic approach to deal with this problem, set up as depicted in **Fig. 1**. A fenestrated bipolar instrument is used in the left arm and a spatula cautery in the right arm to begin dissection. The esophagus is mobilized at the hiatus, and a Penrose is passed around it. Dissection is carefully carried out circumferentially around the esophagus into the chest until the diverticulum is encountered. Using blunt and sharp dissection, the diverticulum is mobilized and the neck dissected. From the assistant port, a stapler is passed through the hiatus along a 60F bougie placed in the esophagus. A vascular stapler is used to minimize leaks from the thin mucosa. The diverticulum is removed for pathologic analysis, and a myotomy is performed on the opposite side of the esophagus extending 2 cm onto the stomach. Because the dissection opens the hiatus, posterior crural sutures of 2-0 Ticron are placed with the bougie in place. Dor fundoplication is then performed.

As with achalasia, the literature addressing the robotic approach to this problem is immature. Two case reports have demonstrated feasibility,[9,10] but further study is required.

Nissen Fundoplication and Giant Paraesophageal Hernia Repair

In the authors' experience, robotic assistance has ameliorated both routine Nissen fundoplication and giant paraesophageal hernia repair (GPEHR). Because the routine antireflux operation is a final component of GPEHR, the authors' approach to this problem is described here. The preoperative workup and operative setup are no different for the robot, and the port placement is as shown in **Fig. 1**. The procedure begins with a fenestrated bipolar instrument in the left arm and a Cadiere in the right arm. With the assistance of a laparoscopic Babcock through the assistant port, the hernia contents are reduced into the abdominal cavity. Endoscopy is performed, and the scope is placed along the greater curvature of the stomach to keep the stomach in the abdomen. The right robot arm instrument is replaced with spatula cautery. The right crus is dissected first, taking great care not to injure its investing peritoneum. The sac is mobilized, and dissection is carried out in the areolar plane between the sac and the mediastinum. The robotic camera is very useful for this maneuver and can be "driven" into the hiatal defect for precise visualization. The sac is reduced into the abdomen, and dissection is carried over to the left crus. The gastroesophageal fat pad is mobilized and resected. The left crus is carefully dissected. Short gastric vessels are divided using the vessel sealer for the robot. A retroesophageal window is created, and a Penrose is placed. At this point, a decision must be made as to whether the esophagus is too short. If 3 cm of esophagus sits in the abdomen without downward retraction, the authors proceed with hiatal repair. If less than 3 cm is visible in the abdomen, the esophagus is mobilized higher into the chest circumferentially. Again, the excellent binocular vision afforded by the robotic camera is extremely useful here. The esophageal length is again assessed. If it is still not adequate, more esophageal mobilization should be performed. Once esophageal mobilization is maximized, if the esophagus is still short then a wedge gastroplasty is performed. A 60F bougie is placed along the lesser curve of the stomach after the endoscope is removed. The fundus of the stomach is folded anteriorly toward the camera, and a 60-mm long linear endoGIA stapler is used to create a staple line from fundus to a point 4 to 6 cm onto the stomach along the bougie (**Fig. 2**). Another staple load is then used from stomach to hiatus, from the end of this staple line to the hiatus along the bougie. The resulting wedge of fundus is removed, and the length of the neo-esophagus is examined. Once enough is sitting in the abdomen without tension, attention is turned to hiatal repair and fundoplication. Bringing the crura together posteriorly is the next step, using interrupted 2-0 Ticron sutures placed with a large suture-cut needle driver in the right arm. A large needle driver in the left arm is used to facilitate tying knots. To facilitate crural apposition, right and left pleural spaces may be entered through the hernia defect to create pneumothoraces and reduce diaphragmatic tension. Rarely, relaxing incisions are necessary. Once the hiatus is closed adequately, a Surgisys overlay mesh is used to buttress the esophageal repair. Attention is then directed to the fundoplication. If the patient has good esophageal function, the authors prefer a complete Nissen, but will perform a Toupet if the patient has extremely poor esophageal motility. The bougie is withdrawn into the

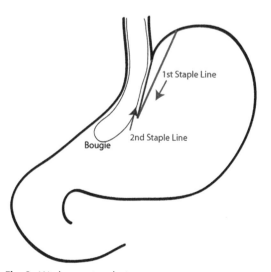

Fig. 2. Wedge gastroplasty.

esophagus, and a fenestrated bipolar instrument is placed in the left robotic arm. This instrument is passed through the retroesophageal widow, and the fundus is grasped. The wrist of the instrument is very helpful in performing this maneuver. The fundus is then brought to the right, and a shoeshine maneuver is performed. At this point, the bougie is carefully replaced into the stomach, and a Nissen (or Toupet) fundoplication is performed using a large suture-cut needle driver in the right arm. A large needle driver in the left arm is used to facilitate tying knots. After the fundoplication is performed, the bougie and all instruments are removed, and all incisions are closed.

Trials comparing laparoscopic Nissen fundoplication with robotic-assisted fundoplication found similar morbidity and postoperative course. The robotic procedures, however, required approximately 30% more time and 55% more cost.[11–14]

Although transthoracic repair of paraesophageal hernia has the best published results,[15] laparoscopic repair has gained favor in the avoidance of thoracotomy.[16–19] However, recurrence rates following laparoscopic repair have been disappointing, with rates of up to 60% in even expert hands.[20] Although robotic assistance will not definitively solve this problem, perhaps the increased visualization and wristed instruments will make this technically demanding operation easier, thereby improving results. However, studies reporting on the efficacy of robot-assisted GPEHR are scarce. Braumann and colleagues[21] described 112 Nissen fundoplications and 14 GPEHRs in 2008, and demonstrated feasibility and safety. Draaisma and colleagues[22] described a prospective case series of 40 patients in which the midterm recurrence rate was low. Finally, Gehrig and colleagues[23] reported a case-control study of 12 robotic, 17 laparoscopic, and 13 open GPEHRs, and not surprisingly noted operative times similar to those of laparoscopic surgery, with similarly low blood loss and hospital stay. Future studies that examine long-term recurrence as well as cost-effectiveness are clearly necessary.

CHEST PROCEDURES
Chest Port Placement

For benign esophageal procedures in the chest, the authors place ports as demonstrated in **Fig. 3**. In general, a 12-mm balloon port is placed in the eighth intercostal space (ICS) posterior to the posterior axillary line. The camera is placed, and 8-mm robot ports are placed in the fifth ICS anteriorly and in the 10th or 11th ICS posteriorly. A 5-mm Step port is placed between the camera

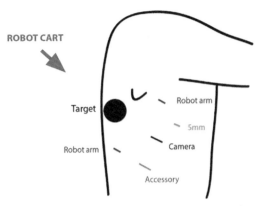

Fig. 3. Port placement for benign esophageal chest procedures.

and right robotic arm port, and a 12-mm Step port is placed between the camera and the left robotic arm port. Insufflation is started at 7 mm Hg.

Robotic Cyst and Benign Mass Excision

Esophageal duplication cysts are congenital anomalies first described by Blasius in 1711. Local surgical resection is recommended to allow for definitive diagnosis and to avoid infectious complications. Traditionally, duplication cysts were resected via a posterolateral thoracotomy. The hypovascular nature of the cysts allowed application of video-assisted thoracoscopic resection early in the technology's evolution.[24,25] The magnification of thoracoscopy aids accurate identification of the vagal and phrenic nerves, and improves the identification of tissue planes. The balance between radical cyst resection and protection of the integrity of esophageal mucosa represents an area where improved visualization of the robot may be beneficial.

Leiomyomas are the most common benign intramural esophageal tumors. Although these tumors produce a characteristic submucosal defect on barium swallow, resection is indicated for definitive diagnosis, as benign esophageal neoplasm only constitutes between 0.5% and 0.8% of all esophageal tumors.[26]

Dissection proceeds with special care, owing to the mobile nature of the esophagus and the machine's lack of haptic feedback. Grasping the cyst or mass with gentle retraction allows careful dissection along the mucosa. The magnification and stereoscopic imaging of the machine is very important. Therefore, the assistant must suction the dissection field when required. The azygous vein is divided, when necessary, using vascular endostaplers. The muscle layer can be closed over the mucosa using techniques identical to

those for open procedures, depending on surgeon preference. After dissection is completed, the cyst is removed in an endocatch bag via the inferior assistant port. If the mucosa is violated, 2-0 Ticron sutures are easily placed in an interrupted fashion using a large suture-cut needle driver in the right arm. A large needle driver in the left arm is used to facilitate knot tying. If necessary to buttress a repair, pleura or even intercostal muscle may be harvested using the excellent vision and wristed instruments.

Published results of robotic approaches to cysts and masses of the esophagus are few. However, the few case reports have demonstrated acceptable operating-room times of between 120 and 150 minutes.[4,27] Again, further study is necessary.

SUMMARY

The application of robotics in surgery does not herald a unique treatment modality but rather the expansion of the tools available for the surgeon. Robotic master-slave devices can assist surgeons to perform minimally invasive esophageal operations with approaches that have already been demonstrated using laparoscopy and thoracoscopy. Robotic techniques and technology should not be viewed as exclusive alternatives to the laparoscopic and thoracoscopic procedures that have demonstrated clinical success.

The advantages and disadvantages of the da Vinci surgical system are still being delineated. Several groups continue to work with robotic technology to improve outcomes and decrease morbidity. Further studies to demonstrate learning curves, assess cost-effectiveness, and evaluate clinical benefit are necessary.

Given the early application of the technology and paucity of clinical evidence, there are currently no procedures for which robotic esophageal surgery is the clinically proven preferred approach. The indications for robotic surgery should closely approximate those for laparoscopic and thoracoscopic procedures. Contraindications are similar to those of other minimally invasive techniques, and are specific to limitations of the robotic device.

REFERENCES

1. Himpens J, Leman G, Cadiere GB. Telesurgical laparoscopic cholecystectomy. Surg Endosc 1998; 12(8):1091.
2. Patti MG, Pellegrini CA, Horgan S, et al. Minimally invasive surgery for achalasia: an 8-year experience with 168 patients. Ann Surg 1999;230(4):587–93 [discussion: 593–4].

3. Luketich JD, Fernando HC, Christie NA, et al. Outcomes after minimally invasive esophagomyotomy. Ann Thorac Surg 2001;72(6):1909–12 [discussion: 1912–3].

4. Giulianotti PC, Coratti A, Angelini M, et al. Robotics in general surgery: personal experience in a large community hospital. Arch Surg 2003;138(7):777–84.

5. Melvin WS, Needleman BJ, Krause KR, et al. Computer-enhanced robotic telesurgery. Initial experience in foregut surgery. Surg Endosc 2002;16(12):1790–2.

6. Zaaijer J. Cardiospasm in the aged. Ann Surg 1923; 77:615–7.

7. Shimi S, Nathanson LK, Cuschieri A. Laparoscopic cardiomyotomy for achalasia. J R Coll Surg Edinb 1991;36(3):152–4.

8. Pellegrini C, Wetter LA, Patti M, et al. Thoracoscopic esophagomyotomy. Initial experience with a new approach for the treatment of achalasia. Ann Surg 1992;216(3):291–6 [discussion: 296–9].

9. Pernazza G, Monsellato I, Pende V, et al. Fully robotic treatment of an epiphrenic diverticulum: report of a case. Minim Invasive Ther Allied Technol 2012; 21(2):96–100.

10. Elola-Olaso AM, Mullett TW, Gagliardi RJ. Epiphrenic diverticulum: robotic-assisted transhiatal approach. Surg Laparosc Endosc Percutan Tech 2009;19(5):184–8.

11. Nguyen NT, Roberts P, Follette DM, et al. Thoracoscopic and laparoscopic esophagectomy for benign and malignant disease: lessons learned from 46 consecutive procedures. J Am Coll Surg 2003; 197(6):902–13.

12. Cadiere GB, Himpens J, Vertruyen M, et al. Evaluation of telesurgical (robotic) NISSEN fundoplication. Surg Endosc 2001;15(9):918–23.

13. Costi R, Himpens J, Bruyns J, et al. Robotic fundoplication: from theoretic advantages to real problems. J Am Coll Surg 2003;197(3):500–7.

14. Melvin WS, Needleman BJ, Krause KR, et al. Computer-enhanced vs. standard laparoscopic antireflux surgery. J Gastrointest Surg 2002;6(1):11–5 [discussion: 15–6].

15. Maziak DE, Todd TR, Pearson FG. Massive hiatus hernia: evaluation and surgical management. J Thorac Cardiovasc Surg 1998;115(1):53–62.

16. Schauer PR, Ikramuddin S, McLaughlin RH, et al. Comparison of laparoscopic versus open repair of paraesophageal hernia. Am J Surg 1998;176(6): 659–65.

17. Velanovich V, Karmy-Jones R. Surgical management of paraesophageal hernia: outcome and quality of life analysis. Dig Surg 2001;18:432–8.

18. Luketich JD, Nason KS, Christie NA, et al. Outcomes after a decade of laparoscopic giant paraesophageal hernia repair. J Thorac Cardiovasc Surg 2010; 139(2):395–404.

19. Antonoff MB, D'Cunha J, Andrade RS, et al. Giant paraesophageal hernia repair: technical pearls. J Thorac Cardiovasc Surg 2012;144(3):S67–70.

20. Oelschlager BK, Pellegrini CA, Hunter JG, et al. Biologic prosthesis to prevent recurrent after laparoscopic paraesophageal hernia repair: long-term follow-up from a multicenter, prospective, randomized trial. J Am Coll Surg 2011;213(4):461–8.

21. Braumann C, Jacobi CA, Menenakos C, et al. Robotic-assisted laparoscopic and thoracoscopic surgery with the da Vinci system: a 4-year experience in a single institution. Surg Laparosc Endosc Percutan Tech 2008;18(3):260–6.

22. Draaisma WA, Gooszen HG, Consten EC, et al. Midterm results of robot-assisted laparoscopic repair of large hiatal hernia: a symptomatic and radiological prospective cohort study. Surg Technol Int 2008; 17:165–70.

23. Gehrig T, Mehrabi A, Fischer L, et al. Robotic-assisted paraesophageal hernia repair—a case-control study. Langenbecks Arch Surg 2013;398(5):691–6.

24. Sugarbaker DJ. Thoracoscopy in the management of anterior mediastinal masses. Ann Thorac Surg 1993;56(3):653–6.

25. Lewis RJ, Caccavale RJ, Sisler GE. Imaged thoracoscopic surgery: a new thoracic technique for resection of mediastinal cysts. Ann Thorac Surg 1992; 53(2):318–20.

26. Orringer MB, Zuidema GD, editors. Surgery of the alimentary tract, vol. 1, 4th edition. Philadelphia: WB Saunders; 1996. p. 369.

27. Elli E, Espat NJ, Berger R, et al. Robotic-assisted thoracoscopic resection of esophageal leiomyoma. Surg Endosc 2004;18(4):713–6.

Index

Note: Page numbers of article titles are in **boldface** type.

Thorac Surg Clin 24 (2014) 231–233
http://dx.doi.org/10.1016/S1547-4127(14)00022-X
1547-4127/14/$ – see front matter © 2014 Elsevier Inc. All rights reserved.

Moving?

Make sure your subscription moves with you!

To notify us of your new address, find your **Clinics Account Number** (located on your mailing label above your name), and contact customer service at:

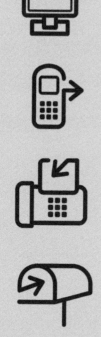

Email: journalscustomerservice-usa@elsevier.com

800-654-2452 (subscribers in the U.S. & Canada)
314-447-8871 (subscribers outside of the U.S. & Canada)

Fax number: 314-447-8029

Elsevier Health Sciences Division
Subscription Customer Service
3251 Riverport Lane
Maryland Heights, MO 63043

*To ensure uninterrupted delivery of your subscription, please notify us at least 4 weeks in advance of move.

Printed and bound by CPI Group (UK) Ltd, Croydon, CR0 4YY

03/10/2024

01040376-0006